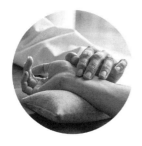

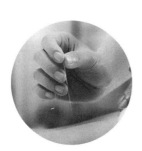

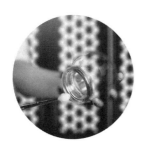

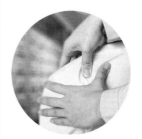

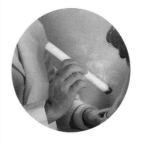

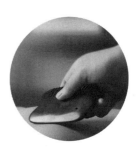

中医养生适宜技术操作规范（海外版）

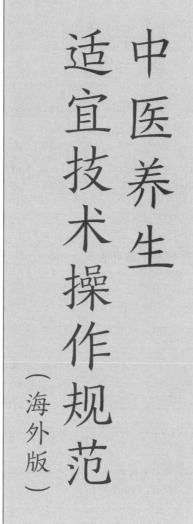

侯江红　吕沛宛　主编

中原农民出版社

·郑州·

图书在版编目（CIP）数据

中医养生适宜技术操作规范：海外版／侯江红，吕沛宛主编 . — 郑州：中原农民出版社，2022.4
ISBN 978－7－5542－2507－3

Ⅰ . ①中… Ⅱ . ①侯… ②吕… Ⅲ . ①养生（中医）- 技术操作规程 Ⅳ . ① R212－65

中国版本图书馆 CIP 数据核字（2021）第 260721 号

中医养生适宜技术操作规范（海外版）
ZHONGYI YANGSHENG SHIYI JISHU CAOZUO GUIFAN（HAIWAIBAN）

出 版 人：刘宏伟
策划策划：刘培英
责任编辑：莫 为 王 铭
责任校对：王艳红
责任印制：孙 瑞
装帧设计：王 婧

出版发行：中原农民出版社
　　　　　地址：郑州市郑东新区祥盛街 27 号　　邮编：450016
　　　　　电话：0371-65788677（编辑部）　　　0371-65713859（发行部）
经　　销：全国新华书店
印　　刷：河南省诚和印制有限公司
开　　本：787mm×1092mm　1/16
印　　张：19.5
字　　数：340 千字
版　　次：2022 年 4 月第 1 版
印　　次：2022 年 4 月第 1 次印刷
定　　价：96.00 元

Contents

中医养生适宜技术操作规范

第一章　中医基础理论

第一节　脏腑学说

脏腑，即人体内脏的总称，包括五脏、六腑和奇恒之腑三类。五脏是指肝、心、脾、肺、肾；六腑指胆、胃、小肠、大肠、膀胱、三焦；奇恒之腑指脑、髓、骨、脉、胆、女子胞。脏与腑的功能特点各有不同，五脏的生理功能是化生和贮藏精、气、血、津液；六腑的生理功能是受纳、腐熟水谷，传化和排泄糟粕；奇恒之腑，异于五脏六腑，因形体上中空有腔与六腑相类，功能上贮藏精气与五脏相同，所以称为奇恒之腑。但其中的胆又属于六腑之一，除"胆"在"六腑"中介绍，女子胞另附"六腑"之后，其他脑、髓、骨、脉均隶属于五脏，分别在"肾""心"二脏内叙述。

脏腑是一个有机的整体。不仅脏与脏、脏与腑、腑与腑在生理、病理上有着密切的联系，而且脏腑与机体组织（筋、脉、肉、皮、骨）和外部器官（鼻、口、舌、目、耳及前后阴）之间有着不可分割的关系。气、血、津液是维持人体生命活动不可缺少的物质，它们的生成、运行和输布，必须通过不同的脏腑功能活动才能完成，而脏腑的各种功能活动，又以气、血、津液作为物质基础。因此，脏腑之间，脏腑与气、血、津液之间，在生理功能和病理变化上都密切相关。

中医学的脏腑和西医学脏器的概念不完全相同。中医学中一个脏腑的功能，可能包括西医学中几个脏器的功能；西医学一个脏器的功能，可能分散在中医学几个脏腑的功能之中。这是因为脏腑在中医学里不单纯是一个解剖学的概念，更重要的是一个生理或病理学方面的概念，例如脏腑中的"心"，除了代表解剖学上的实体外，还包括了精神、思维活动的功能。因此，不能把中医学的脏腑功能和西医学的脏器等同起来。

一、五脏

（一）肝

肝位于腹腔，横膈之下，右胁之内。它的主要功能是主疏泄，主藏血。

1. **主疏泄** 疏泄，是疏通宣泄的意思。肝主疏泄，是指肝对人体的气机有疏通宣泄的功能。疏泄功能主要体现在两个方面：

（1）情志方面：肝有调节情志活动的功能。人的精神情志活动，除了由心所主之外，与肝的关系也很密切，只有肝的疏泄功能正常，气机通畅，才能气血平和，心情舒畅。如肝失疏泄，气机失调，就可以引起情志的异常变化，肝气抑郁，则见胸胁胀满、闷闷不乐、多疑善虑等症；肝气亢盛，则见急躁易怒、失眠多梦、头胀头痛、目眩头晕等症。

（2）消化方面：肝的疏泄功能，一方面可以通调气机，助脾胃之气的升降，是保证脾胃正常消化功能的重要条件；另一方面可以促进胆汁的分泌，有助于水谷的消化。如果肝失疏泄，也常影响到脾胃的消化功能，出现嗳气、呕吐、恶心、腹痛、腹泻等症，称"肝气犯胃"和"肝脾不和"。

2. **主藏血** 肝主藏血是指肝具有贮藏血液和调节血量的功能。血液在人体内常随着不同的生理活动而改变。当人体在活动的时候，血液趋向活动的组织器官肝脏将贮藏的血液输出，以供给机体；休息和睡眠时，大量的血液又归藏于肝。

3. **主筋，"其华在爪"** 筋即筋膜，是一种联络关节、肌肉的组织。肝主筋，是指全身的筋膜依赖肝血的滋养。肝血充盈，筋膜得到充分濡养，才能维持其正常功能。如果肝血不足，血不养筋，则可出现肢体麻木、屈伸不利，甚至手足震颤、四肢抽搐。肝血的盛衰可以影响到爪甲的荣枯变化。

4. **开窍于目** "肝开窍于目"，是指肝的经脉上连目系。目得肝血的濡养才能发挥正常的视觉功能。

（二）心

心位于胸中，有心包络围护于外。它的主要功能是主血脉，主神志。

1. **主血脉，"其华在面"** 心主血脉，是指心脏有推动血液在脉管内运行以营养全身的功能，所以说"心主身之血脉"。心脏之所以能推动血液的运行，主要是依赖心气的作用。心气旺盛，就能使血液在脉管中运行不息，以满足全身的需要。由于血液在脉管中运行，而面部的血脉又比较丰富，所以心气的盛衰，可以从脉搏的变化和面部色泽反映出来。若心气旺盛，血脉充盈，则脉搏和缓有力，面色红润而有光泽，就是所说的"其华在面"；若心气不足，血脉空虚，则面色白而无光泽。

2. **主神志**　神志是指人的精神、意识、思维活动。根据现代生理学的认识，精神、意识、思维活动，是大脑的功能，即大脑对外界客观事物的反应。中医学认为神志与五脏有关，而主要属于心的生理功能。若心血不足，常出现心烦、失眠、多梦、健忘、神志不宁等症。

3. **开窍于舌**　心与舌在生理上密切相关。心的经络上系于舌，其气血上通于舌。如果心有病变，就容易从舌体上反映出来。

（三）脾

脾位于中焦。它的主要功能是主运化，统摄血液。

1. **主运化**　脾主运化的功能包括两个方面：

（1）运化水谷精微：主要是指脾有消化食物和吸收、运输营养物质的功能。食物入胃，经过胃与脾的共同消化，其中的水谷精微通过脾气输布全身，以营养五脏六腑、四肢百骸，以及皮毛、筋肉等组织。由于饮食水谷是人出生后所需营养物质的主要来源，也是生成气血的主要物质基础，所以脾被称为"后天之本"和"气血生化之源"。如果脾气健运，则消化、吸收、输布功能旺盛；若脾失健运，则会引起腹胀、便溏、食欲不振、倦怠、消瘦等病症。

（2）运化水液：脾有调节水液代谢的作用，在与肺、肾的共同作用下，来维持人体水液正常的代谢。若脾失健运，可引起痰饮、水肿等水湿潴留的病症。

2. **主肌肉、四肢**　是由于脾具有运化水谷精微的功能，使肌肉、四肢得到供养。脾气健运，营养供应充足，则肌肉丰满，四肢轻劲、灵活有力。脾失健运，营养缺乏，则肌肉消瘦或痿弱，四肢倦怠无力。

3. **主统血**　统是统摄、控制的意思。脾主统血，是指脾气有统摄血液，使血液循环于脉道之中而不溢出脉道的功能。如果脾气虚弱，失去统摄的功能，血液就会溢出脉道，出现便血、崩漏、肌衄等病症。

4. **开窍于口，其华在唇**　脾开窍于口指人的饮食、口味与脾的运化功能密切相关，口唇的变化能反映出脾气的盛衰。脾气健运则饮食旺盛，口味正常，口唇红润有光泽。脾失健运则不思饮食，口淡乏味，口唇萎黄不泽。所以说脾"开窍于口，其华在唇"。

（四）肺

肺位于胸腔，左右各一，覆盖于心之上。它的主要功能是主气，司呼吸，主宣发、肃降，朝百脉，主治节。

1. **主气，司呼吸**　肺主气包括两个方面：

（1）主呼吸之气：肺脏有司呼吸的作用，是机体内外气体交换的场所。人体通过肺的呼吸，吸入自然界的清气，呼出体内的浊气，使体内外的气体不断得到交换。《素问·阴阳应象大论》说的"天气通于肺"，就是这个意思。

（2）主一身之气：这是因为肺与宗气的生成密切相关。宗气是由水谷之精气与肺所吸入的清气结合而成的，积于胸中，又通过心脉散布全身，以维持机体的正常生理活动。

肺主气的功能正常，则气道通畅，呼吸均匀。若肺气不足，不仅呼吸功能减弱，而且会影响宗气的生成，出现呼吸无力、气短、语音低微等气虚症状。

2. **主宣发、肃降**　肺的宣发与肃降是相辅相成的两个方面。肺有宣有降，才能呼吸调匀、水道通畅，保持水液的正常运行和输布。

（1）主宣发，外合皮毛：宣发，是宣布、发散的意思，即向上向外布散气和津液。肺主宣发，是指由于肺气的推动，使卫气和津液布散全身，以温润肌腠皮毛。皮毛位于体表，是人体抵御外邪侵袭的屏障。皮毛由肺输布的卫气与津液所温养，所以肺与皮毛在生理上关系密切，病理上也相互影响。若肺气虚弱，不能宣发卫气和津液于皮毛，不仅可使皮毛憔悴、枯槁，还可导致卫气不固，易感外邪。

（2）主肃降，通调水道：肃降是清肃下降的意思，即向下向内散布气和津液。肺的位置在上焦，肺气则以清肃下降为顺。若肺气不能正常地肃降，就会出现胸闷、咳嗽、喘息等肺气上逆的病症。同时，肺气的肃降，可以使上焦的水液不断地下输到肾和膀胱，保持着小便的通利。

3. **朝百脉，主治节**　肺朝百脉，是指全身的血液通过百脉，流经于肺，经肺的呼吸进行气体交换，然后再将新的血液输送到全身。肺主治节，是指肺具有调节呼吸和全身气、血、津液、水液的作用。若肺气充沛，则血运正常，气机通畅。若肺气虚弱，则心血不行，血脉瘀滞，出现心悸、舌紫等症状。

4. **开窍于鼻**　鼻的通气和嗅觉的功能，主要依靠肺气的作用。肺气和，则鼻窍通利、嗅觉灵敏。若外邪袭肺，肺气不宣，则出现鼻塞流涕、嗅觉不灵敏等病症；肺热壅盛，则出现喘促、鼻翼扇动等病症，所以称"鼻为肺窍"。

（五）肾

肾位于腰部脊柱两侧，左右各一。它的主要功能是藏精，主水液，主纳气。

1. **藏精** 是指肾主人体的生长发育、生殖和脏腑气化。肾脏所藏的精包括先天之精和后天之精两个方面。先天之精受之于父母，是人体生长发育、繁殖的基本物质。后天之精，来源于饮食精微，由脾胃化生，是维持人体生命活动的基本物质。先天之精与后天之精是相互依存、相互促进的。先天之精必须有后天之精的供养，才能得到不断的充实；后天之精又必须依赖先天之精才能化生。

精能化气，肾精所化之气，称为肾气。肾气由肾精化生，分为肾阴和肾阳，能够促进人体生长发育和生殖。从幼年开始，肾的精气逐渐充盛；到青春期，肾气充盈，性功能逐渐成熟，而有生育能力；到了老年，肾的精气渐衰，性功能和生殖能力随之减退而至消失，形体也逐渐衰老。这一过程反映了肾的精气在人体生长发育和生殖方面的作用。如小儿发育迟缓以及某些不孕症都是肾的精气不足的表现。

2. **主水液** 是指肾有主司和调节人体水液代谢的功能。人体水液代谢与肺、脾、肾三脏有关，但主要是肾的气化作用。在正常的情况下，水液经过胃的受纳、脾的转输、肺的输布，并通过三焦将水液中清的部分运送到全身各脏腑，浊的部分化为小便排出体外，使体内水液代谢维持着相对平衡。这些作用的发挥，都有赖于肾阳的蒸化。如果肾的气化失常，就会出现小便不利、水肿等水液代谢障碍的病症。

3. **主纳气** 人体的呼吸功能虽然是肺所主，但肾又有摄纳肺气的作用，即帮助肺脏吸气，使吸入之气下达于肾，只有肾气充足，摄纳正常，才能使肺的气道通畅、呼吸均匀。如肾气虚，出现呼吸困难、动则气喘等病症，称为"肾不纳气"。

4. **主骨、生髓、通于脑，其华在发** 肾藏精，精能生髓，髓藏于骨中，充养骨骼，所以肾精是生长骨骼的物质基础。肾精充足，则骨髓的生化有源，骨骼得到滋养而坚强有力。若肾精亏虚，骨髓的生化之源不足，不能充养骨骼，便会出现骨骼软弱无力、骨质疏松、发育不良等病症。所以，小儿囟门迟闭、骨软无力，多由先天肾精不足所致。

髓有骨髓和脊髓之分。脊髓上通于脑，脑为髓聚而成，所以称"脑为髓之海"。人的精神活动主要为心所主，但与脑密切相关，明代李时珍称"脑为元神之府"。因为脑髓依赖肾精才能不断生化，所以人的精神活动也与肾的功能有关。

发的润养来源于血，故称头发为"血余"。但头发还需肾精的充养。因此，头发的生长与脱落、润泽与枯槁，都与肾精的盛衰有关。青壮年肾精充足，头发乌黑致密有光泽；老年人肾气虚衰，则头发变白而易脱落。

5. 开窍于耳，司二便　耳的听觉功能，依赖于肾的精气充养。若肾气充足，则听觉灵敏。若肾精不足，则出现耳鸣、听力减退等症。老年人多见耳聋失聪，往往是肾精亏虚的缘故。

尿液的贮存和排泄虽在膀胱，但要依赖肾的气化。若肾虚气化失常，则出现小便不利；若肾虚不固，则见小便失禁或遗尿。大便的排泄也要受肾气影响及控制，肾阳虚衰可致大便秘结，肾气不固可致久泄滑脱。

二、六腑

（一）胆

胆附于肝，储藏胆汁，胆汁促进食物的消化和吸收。若肝胆之气不能疏泄下行，或湿热熏蒸肝胆，则可见口苦、呕吐苦水或一身、面目发黄等胆气上逆、胆汁外溢的病症。胆虽为六腑之一，但它储藏精汁而不接受水谷或糟粕，与其他五脏有所不同，故又把它归属于"奇恒之腑"。

（二）胃

胃位于膈下，上接食管，下通小肠。胃的主要生理功能是受纳、腐熟水谷。饮食入口，经过食管，容纳于胃，所以称胃为"水谷之海"。容纳在胃中的水谷经过胃的腐熟消磨，下传小肠，其中精微物质通过脾的运化以供养周身，这种功能又称为"胃气"。胃气的盛衰不仅影响胃肠的功能活动，而且对其他脏腑也有一定的影响。中医学一向重视"胃气"的作用，因为胃是受纳、腐熟水谷，供给营养物质的重要器官，所以说"人以胃气为本"。对于病情的观察也非常重视胃的功能状况，认为"有胃气则生，无胃气则死"，以此作为判断疾病预后的一个重要方面。

（三）小肠

小肠上接胃，下通大肠。它的主要功能是泌别清浊。小肠将胃传下来的水谷进一步加以消化，并把它分成清、浊两部分，其中清的部分由脾输送到全身，浊的部分通过阑门下注大肠，过剩的水液则渗入膀胱。所以，食物的消化、吸收和大小便的排泄都与小肠有密切的关系。若小肠有病，除影响消化吸收功能外，还会出现大小便异常。

（四）大肠

大肠上接小肠，下端为肛门，主要功能是传化糟粕。大肠接受小肠下注的浊物，吸收其中多余的水分，使食物残渣成为粪便，由肛门排出体外。若大肠有病则致传化失常，出现便秘、痢疾、腹胀、腹泻等病症。

（五）膀胱

膀胱位于下腹。它的主要功能是贮存和排泄尿液。膀胱是主持水液代谢的器官之一，水液通过脾、肺、肾、三焦诸脏腑的作用布散全身，代谢后的水分经三焦水道下达膀胱成为尿液，并通过膀胱的气化功能排出体外。若膀胱气化失常，可出现小便不利、癃闭等病症；若膀胱失去约束，可见尿频、小便失禁等病症。

（六）三焦

三焦是上焦、中焦、下焦的总称。三焦虽属六腑之一，但一般认为它并不是一个独立的脏器，而是包含了胸腹腔上、中、下三部有关的脏腑及其部分功能。从部位来分，胃脘部相当于中焦，以上为上焦，以下为下焦。从内脏来说，上焦包括心、肺；中焦包括脾、胃，下焦包括肝、肾、膀胱等脏器。

附：女子胞

女子胞又名胞宫，位于小腹，属奇恒之腑，有主月经和孕育胎儿的作用。

三、脏腑之间的关系

（一）脏与脏

1. **心与肺**　心主血，肺主气，心肺两脏互相配合，才能保证气血的正常运行。若肺气虚弱，推动心血无力，血运不畅，日久则形成心血瘀阻，出现胸闷、气短、心悸、唇青、舌紫等病症。若心主血的功能减退，血液运行不畅，也会影响肺的宣降功能，而出现咳嗽、喘息等症。

2. **心与肾**　心居于上，肾居于下，两者功能主要在于心阳和肾水之间的平衡。若肾水不足，不能上滋心阴，就会出现心悸、心烦、失眠等病症；若心阳不振，心火不能下温肾阳，就会出现心悸、心慌、水肿等病症。

3. **心与脾**　心主血，脾统血。脾的功能健旺，则血液生化之源充足，而心血充盈。血液运行于经脉之中，既赖心气的推动，又需要脾气的统摄。心脾两脏相互配合，才能保证血液的不断生成和正常运行。若脾失健运，会导致血的化源不足；若脾不统血，可导致心血不足；若思虑过度，耗损心血，又能影响脾的健运，常形成心脾两虚的证候。

4.肝与肾 肝藏血，肾藏精。肝血有赖于肾精的滋养，肾精也需要肝血所化之精的补充。由于精与血相互资生，所以有"精血同源""肝肾同源"的说法。

5.脾与肾 脾为后天之本，肾为先天之本。脾的运化功能需要肾阳温煦功能的辅助；肾的先天精气又必须依赖后天水谷精微的补充。脾与肾，是相互资助，相互促进的。

6.肝与脾 肝主疏泄，脾主运化，两者生理上密切相关，病理上相互影响。脾胃的升降、运化，依赖肝气的疏泄。肝的疏泄正常，才能使脾胃升降适度，运化健全。若两者关系不均衡，则会出现胸胁胀满、嗳气、呕吐、腹痛、腹泻等病症。

（二）脏与腑

脏与腑，主要是表里相合的关系。脏属阴，腑属阳；阳主表，阴主里。脏腑之间，通过经脉的相互络属，构成表里关系。表里之间在生理上相互配合，病理上也相互影响。分别介绍如下：

1.心与小肠 心与小肠相表里。心与小肠的关系表现在病理方面较为明显。若心经实火，可"移热于小肠"，出现尿少、尿赤、排尿灼热等病症；若小肠有热，也可以循经脉上熏于心，出现心烦、舌赤或糜烂等病症。

2.肺与大肠 肺与大肠相表里。肺气肃降，则大肠的传导功能才能正常；而大肠传导通畅，又有助于肺气的肃降。若肺失肃降，影响大肠的传导，可导致大便困难、腹胀等病症；若大肠壅滞不通，又可以引起肺气不降，出现咳喘、胸满等病症。

3.脾与胃 脾与胃相表里。脾主运化，胃主受纳。脾气以升为顺，胃气以降为和。脾气上升，水谷精气才能上输；胃气下降，饮食水谷才能下行。脾属阴，喜燥恶湿；胃属阳，喜润恶燥。脾胃脏腑阴阳相合，升降相因，燥湿相济，互相协调，共同完成食物的消化、吸收以及水谷精气的运输、布散。

4.肝与胆 胆附于肝，肝与胆相表里。肝的疏泄功能正常，保证了胆汁的排泄通畅；胆汁排泄正常，又有助于肝的疏泄，因此两者密切相关。肝胆在病理上也相互影响，常出现肝胆同病，如肝胆火旺、肝胆湿热等证候。

5.肾与膀胱 肾与膀胱相表里。膀胱的气化功能与肾气密切相关。若肾气充足，膀胱气化功能正常，开合有度，能保持正常的贮尿和排尿功能；若肾气不足，气化失职，膀胱开合失常，就可出现小便不利或失禁、遗尿、尿频等病症。所以有关尿液的贮存与排泄的病变，除膀胱本身外，多与肾脏有关。

（三）腑与腑

六腑的主要功能是传导化物，它们相互协作，共同完成食物的消化、吸收和排泄的全过程。饮食入胃，经胃的腐熟，下降于小肠，胆排泄胆汁入肠以助消化；小肠承受胃腐熟的水谷，再进一步消化，并泌别清浊，清的部分作为营养供应全身，浊的部分进入大肠，水液渗入膀胱；进入大肠的糟粕，经过大肠的再吸收，将废物（粪便）排出体外；水液渗入膀胱而化为尿液，经气化作用排出体外；而在整个消化、吸收和排泄的过程中，又有赖于三焦的气化、疏通水道的作用。

以上可以看出六腑在生理上的密切关系。六腑在病理上也相互影响，一腑有病变可以涉及他腑。如胃有实热，消灼津液，可使大便燥结，大肠传导不利；肠燥便闭，又可影响胃的和降，使胃气上逆，出现恶心、呕吐等病症。

第二节　经络与经络系统

一、经络

经络是人体组织结构的重要组成部分。它遍布全身，使内部脏腑和外部各组织器官联系成为一个有机的整体。它是人体运行气血的通路。

经络学说是中医基础理论的重要组成部分。长期以来它一直指导着中医各科的临床实践，尤其在针灸、推拿等方面，有着十分重要的意义。近年来，根据经络学说的理论，发展了不少新疗法，如针刺麻醉、水针疗法、埋线疗法及穴位结扎疗法等，从而丰富了经络学说的内容。

1. **经络的概念**　经络是经脉和络脉的总称。经，有"路径"的意思。经脉是经络中直行的主干，如十二经脉。络，有"网络"的意思。络脉是经脉的分支，有别络、浮络及孙络之分。它们纵横交错，网络全身，无处不至。

经络是运行全身气血、联络周身表里、沟通上下内外、调节体内各部分的通路。通过经络遍布全身，把人体的五脏六腑、四肢百骸、五官九窍、皮肉筋骨等组织器官联结成为一个有机的整体。

2. **经络的组成**　经络是由经脉和络脉组成的。经脉分为十二正经和奇经八脉两大类，为经络系统的主要部分。十二正经即太阴、少阴、厥阴三阴经和太阳、少阳、阳明三阳经，六经手足各一，合称"十二经脉"。奇经八脉，即督脉、任脉、冲脉、带脉、阴跷脉、阳跷脉、阴维脉和阳维脉。络脉分为别络、浮络和孙络。别络较大，共有十五，即十二正经和督、任二脉各有一支别络，再加上脾之大络，合为"十五别络"。络脉浮行在浅表部位的称"浮络"。络脉最细小的分支称为"孙络"。

此外，还有十二经别、十二经筋和十二皮部等。

3. 经络的作用

（1）生理方面：经络有沟通表里上下、联络脏腑器官、运行气血、抗御外邪、保卫机体的作用。人体的五脏六腑、四肢九窍、皮肉筋骨等组织器官，各有不同的生理功能，但使机体保持着协调统一，构成有机的统一整体。这种相互联系，有机配合，主要是依靠经络系统的沟通作用来实现。同时，经络又是运行气血的通路，在心气的推动下，使气血周流全身，以营养各组织器官，并发挥抗御外邪、保卫机体的作用，从而维持人体正常的生理活动。

（2）病理方面：经络在病理上主要是与疾病的发生和传变密切相关。当人体正气不足，经络失去正常的机能时，就容易遭受外邪的侵袭而发病。疾病发生后，病邪常沿着经络自外而内、由表入里的传变。因此，经络在生理上是运行气血的通路，在病理上又是疾病发展传变的通路。

经络不仅是外邪由表入里的传变途径，而且也是脏腑之间、脏腑与体表组织器官之间病变相互影响的重要渠道。通过经络的联系，脏腑病变可以相互影响，如肝病影响胃，心病移热于小肠等；内脏病变可以反映到体表的一定部位，如胃火的牙龈肿痛，肝火的目赤肿痛，胆火的耳聋、耳痛等病症。

（3）诊断方面：经络内属脏腑，并在体表有固定的循行部位，因此，内脏病变可以在有关的经脉上反映出来。临床上常根据疾病所出现的症状，结合经络的循行部位及其所属（络）的脏腑，来诊断疾病。如两胁疼痛多肝胆疾病；腰痛多属肾病等。不同脏腑的病变，也可以在所属经络的某些穴位上出现反应，如肺脏有病，在中府穴有压痛点；阑尾炎在阑尾穴有压痛点等。此外，经络的循行分布规律，也可作为某些疾病诊断的依据。如头痛一症，前额痛属阳明经；两侧头痛属少阳经；头项痛属太阳经；头顶痛属厥阴经等。

（4）治疗方面：经络学说广泛地应用于临床各科的治疗，特别是对针灸、按摩和药物治疗，都具有重要的指导意义。

在药物治疗方面，由于某些药物对某些脏腑经络有特殊的治疗作用，因而产生了"药物归经"的理论，对临床用药有一定的指导作用。如羌活、白芷、柴胡三药同样可以治头痛，羌活治疗太阳头痛，白芷治疗阳明头痛，柴胡治疗少阳头痛。又如黄连、黄芩、黄柏三药都能清热，而黄连善于清心热，黄芩善于清肺热，黄柏善于清肾热等。

在针灸治疗方面，也常用循经取穴的方法以治疗某一脏腑组织的病症。如胃痛，取胃经的足三里；如肝病，刺肝经的期门等。当前被广泛用于外科临床的针刺麻醉术，也是在经络学说的理论基础上发展起来的，是通过针刺一定的经穴以达到麻醉镇痛作用的。

其他如推拿、气功等疗法也广泛地应用经络理论。

二、十二经脉

（一）十二经脉的命名

十二经脉的命名，是以经脉所属脏腑的名称和循行的主要部位，并结合阴阳理论而定的。如联属心脏的经脉称为"心经"，联属肺脏的经脉称为"肺经"。主要循行在上肢的经脉称"手经"，主要循行在下肢的经脉称"足经"。与脏相联者为"阴经"，与腑相联者为"阳经"。如手太阴肺经，是指这一经脉循行在上肢，属肺，肺是五脏之一，属阴。

十二经脉名称分类表

性属及循行 手足	阴经 （属脏）	阳经 （属腑）	主要循行部位 阴经行内侧，阳经行外侧	
手	太阴肺经	阳明大肠经	上肢	前线
	厥阴心包经	少阳三焦经		中线
	少阴心经	太阳小肠经		后线
足	太阴脾经	阳明胃经	下肢	前线
	厥阴肝经	少阳胆经		中线
	少阴肾经	太阳膀胱经		后线

注：在小腿下半部和足背部，肝经在前线，脾经在中线。在内踝尖上8寸处交叉后，脾经在前线，肝经在中线。

（二）十二经脉的走向、交接、分布规律及流注次序

1. 走向、交接和分布规律　十二经脉即手三阴经，手三阳经，足三阳经，足三

阴经。它们的走向、交接和分布的规律是：手三阴经，从胸走手，交手三阳经；手三阳经，从手走头，交足三阳经；足三阳经，从头走足，交足三阴经；足三阴经，从足走腹，交手三阴经。

从以上的规律可以看出，阳经与阳经交接于头面；阴经与阴经交接于胸腹；阴经与阳经交接于四肢末端。

阴经分布在四肢的内侧，其排列次序是：太阴经在前，厥阴经居中，少阴经在后；下肢内侧，内踝尖上八寸以下是厥阴在前，太阴在中，少阴在后。阳经分布在四肢外侧，其排列次序是：阳明经在前，少阳经居中，太阳经在后。

2. **表里关系及流注次序** 十二经脉内系六脏（包括心包络）、六腑，构成了六对阴阳表里相合的经脉关系。手太阴肺经与手阳明大肠经相表里；手少阴心经与手太阳小肠经相表里；手厥阴心包经与手少阳三焦经相表里；足太阴脾经与足阳明胃经相表里；足少阴肾经与足太阳膀胱经相表里；足厥阴肝经与足少阳胆经相表里。它们的表里关系体现在两个方面：一是脏腑相互络属，阴经属脏络腑，阳经属腑络脏。二是四肢末端表里交接，手的阴经交阳经，足的阳经交阴经。由于手足阴阳十二经脉存在着这种表里关系，所以在生理上彼此相通，病理上又相互影响。

十二经脉分布在人体内外，气血在经脉中的运行是循环贯注的，即从手太阴肺经开始，依次传至足厥阴肝经，再传到手太阴肺经。如此循环，周流不息。十二经脉流注次序如下：手太阴肺经→手阳明大肠经→足阳明胃经→足太阴脾经→手少阴心经→手太阳小肠经→足太阳膀胱经→足少阴肾经→手厥阴心包经→手少阳三焦经→足少阳胆经→足厥阴肝经→手太阴肺经。

（三）奇经八脉

奇经八脉即督脉、任脉、冲脉、带脉、阴跷脉、阳跷脉、阴维脉、阳维脉。由于它们多与脏腑没有直接的联系，又没有表里配合关系，不同于十二正经，故称"奇经"。奇经八脉交叉贯穿于十二经脉之间，有加强经脉之间联系、调节十二经脉气血的作用。现将其中与临床关系较密切的督、任、冲、带四脉介绍如下。

1. **督脉** 督脉有总督一身阳经的作用。十二经脉中的手足三阳经脉均会于督脉，所以又称督脉为"阳脉之海"。

2. **任脉** 任脉有总任一身阴经的作用，故称任脉为"阴脉之海"。任，还有妊养的意思，其脉起于胞中，在女子具有孕育胎儿的作用，所以又有"任主胞胎"的说法。

3. **冲脉**　冲脉有总管全身气血的功能，为一身气血的要冲，故冲脉有"十二经之海"和"血海"之称。

4. **带脉**　带脉起于季胁，围绕腰腹一周，状如束带，故名带脉。带脉有总束阴阳经脉的作用，所以有"诸脉皆属于带"的说法。带脉不和，多见妇女带下诸病。

（四）背俞穴的独特应用

足太阳膀胱经，从眼内角睛明穴起始，上行至额，再上与督脉在巅顶相交，从头顶深行入脑，还出下行，并沿肩胛内侧，挟行于脊柱两旁，是背部经脉的主要干线之一，共有十八对俞穴。背俞穴是脏腑之气输注于背部的特定腧穴，其所在部位与本脏腑相近，能反映脏腑病症，可以用来治疗内脏病症。

（五）五脏俞加膈俞

所谓俞穴，系指脏腑经气输注于背部的腧穴。也就是说，脏腑的经气都输注于此，诸凡脏腑的气血之盛衰，在其相应的俞穴部位均可表现出来。

足太阳膀胱经在表属阳，五脏在里属阴《素问·阴阳应象大论》"善用针者，从阴引阳，从阳引阴，以右治左，以左治右，以我知彼，以表知里，以观过与不及之理，见微得过，用之不殆"，所谓"从阴引阳，从阳引阴"之意，张志聪注曰："夫阴阳、气血、外内、左右交相贯通，故善用针者，从阴而引阳分之邪，从阳而引阴分之气。"

五脏俞之中，肺俞位置最高，在第三胸椎下缘，正中旁开一寸半。肺主一身之气，司呼吸又主皮毛，司腠理之开合，外邪入侵，肺卫首当其冲，肺气虚则肺俞不满，针刺肺俞，既可宣通肺气、清热和营，又能补益肺气、理气调气。心俞在第五胸椎下缘，旁开一寸半。心主血而藏神，心气心血不足则心俞不满，针刺心俞则有理血和营、安神宁心之功。肝俞在第九胸椎下缘，旁开一寸半。肝藏血，主疏泄，喜条达，主筋，肝气横逆犯胃，肝不藏血则血溢衄血，肝血虚则肝俞不满，针刺肝俞则有舒肝解郁、和血安神之功。脾俞在十一胸椎下缘，旁开一寸半。脾主运化，主统血，脾虚不运则消化机能出现障碍，脾与胃相表里，脾升胃降，上下通调，气机舒畅，中焦堵塞则升降失司，脾虚则脾俞不满，针脾俞则有健脾利湿、和胃调中、调理升降之功。肾俞在第二腰椎棘突下，旁开一寸半。肾藏精，主命门火，为人体元阴元阳之所在。《景岳全书》说："命门为精血之海，脾胃为水谷之海，均为五脏六腑之本；然命门为元气之根，为水火之宅，五脏之阴气，非此不能滋；五脏之阳气，非此不能发；而脾胃以中央之土，非火不能生。"肾虚则五脏之精气不藏，命门之火衰则五脏六腑之阳气无以发，肾俞不满，针刺肾俞则有培补肾气、填精益阴之功。五脏之间相生相克，功能协调则生机旺盛，五脏不和则百病始生。

膈俞在足太阳膀胱经十八对俞穴中，为八会穴之一，亦即"血会膈俞"。针刺膈俞则有理血调气、升清降浊、疏通气血、统治一切血病之功。所以，五脏俞加膈俞的总体功能是坚固五脏、调气和血、扶正固本、调理阴阳。

第三节　中医诊法的操作常规

诊法，是诊察疾病的方法。包括望诊、闻诊、问诊、切诊四个内容，又称为"四诊"。在诊察疾病时，必须认真细致，"四诊合参"。从整体观念出发，了解疾病显现于外在的症状和体征，以推断疾病的原因、性质及其内部联系，从而对疾病做出全面的分析和正确的判断，为辨证论治提供可靠的依据。

一、望诊

望诊，是指对患者的精神、面色、形态、舌象等进行有目的的观察，以了解其疾病情况的一种诊察方法，包括望全身情况和望局部情况。在医疗实践中，人们逐渐认识到人体脏腑气血阴阳的某些变化，能从人体外部，特别是面部和舌部反映出来。因此，通过望诊就可了解机体内部的某些病变。

（一）望全身情况

1. 望神　神，指人体生命活动总的外在表现，又指人的精神、意识思维活动。神是以精气作为物质基础的。望神，主要是通过观察患者的精神状态、意识活动、语言气息，来判断脏腑气血阴阳的盛衰和疾病的轻重及预后。

一般来说，精气盛则神旺，精气衰则神疲。如患者两眼灵活、明亮有神、神志清楚、语言清晰、反应灵敏者，称为"有神"或"得神"，表示正气未伤、病情轻浅、预后良好；若目光晦暗、瞳神呆滞、精神萎靡、语言低微、反应迟钝，甚至神志昏迷、循衣摸床、撮空理线者，则称为"无神"或"失神"，表示正气已伤，病情较重，预后较差。

2. 望面色　是指观察面部的颜色与光泽。面部的色泽是脏腑气血的外部反映。所以，望面色可以推断病情变化的情况。

3. 望形体　是指通过观察患者形体的强、弱、胖、瘦等情况，以了解体质的强弱和内脏气血的盛衰。凡形体结实、骨骼粗大、胸廓宽厚、肌肉充实、皮肤润泽者，是气血充盛的表现；而形体瘦弱、骨骼细小、胸廓狭窄、肌肉瘦削、皮肤枯槁，是气血虚衰的表现。

4. **望姿态** 是指观察患者的动静姿态以及与疾病有关的体位变化，以测知内在疾病的诊察方法。不同的疾病可使人出现不同的姿态和体位。如患者喜动多言，多属阳证；患者喜静少言，多属阴证。若患者身轻能自转侧，面常向外，多为阳证、热证、实证；若身重难于转侧，面常向里，多为阴证、寒证、虚证；若患者卧时仰面伸足，揭去衣被，不欲近火者，多属热证；若卧时蜷缩成团，喜加衣被或向火取暖者，多属寒证。

（二）望局部情况

1. **望头和发** 是指通过望患者的头和发以了解肾和气血的盛衰情况。

小儿头形过大或过小，伴智力不全，多属肾精亏损；囟门下陷，多为虚证；囟门高突，多属热证；囟门迟闭，头项软弱者，多为肾气不足。

发稀疏易落，或干枯不荣，多为精血不足；突然出现片状脱发，多属血虚受风。

2. **望目** 目为肝之窍，但五脏六腑之精气皆上注于目，故目的病变不仅与肝相关，也可反映其他脏腑的病变。如目赤红肿，多属风热或肝火；白睛发黄，多为黄疸；目眦淡白，属气血不足；目眦赤烂，多属湿热；目胞浮肿，多为水肿；目窝下陷，多为津液亏耗。

3. **望口唇** 应观察其颜色、润燥和形态的变化。如口唇淡白，多属血虚；唇色青紫，为寒凝血瘀；唇深红而干，为热盛伤津；唇色鲜红，为阴虚火旺；口唇糜烂，为脾胃蕴热；口角㖞斜，多为中风。

4. **望齿、龈** 齿乃骨之余，龈为胃之络。应注意其色泽和局部的变化。如牙齿干燥，多为胃热炽盛；牙齿松动稀疏、齿根外露者，多属肾虚或虚火上炎；睡中咬牙，多为食积或虫积；牙龈色白，多为血虚；牙龈红肿疼痛，多为胃火上炎。

5. **望咽喉** 应注意其颜色及形态的异常改变。如咽喉红肿而痛，多属肺胃蕴热；咽喉红肿溃烂、有黄白腐点，多为肺胃热毒壅盛；咽喉红色娇嫩，不甚疼痛，多为阴虚火旺；咽喉如有灰白膜，擦之不去、重剥则出血、随即复生者，是为白喉。

6. **望斑疹** 应注意其色泽和形态的变化。皮下出现红色片状斑块，压之不褪色、摸之不碍手者，称为"斑"。若皮下出现红色疹点，小如粟粒、摸之碍手、压之色褪者，称为"疹"。

（三）望舌

望舌，又称"舌诊"，是中医望诊中的重要部分。脏腑的病变可通过舌象反映出来。

望舌，主要是观察舌质和舌苔两个方面。舌质，也称舌体，是舌的肌肉脉络组织。舌苔，由胃气所生，是附着于舌面上的一层苔状物。正常舌象：舌体柔软、活动自如、颜色淡红，舌面上铺有颗粒均匀、干湿适中的薄白苔。一般称为"淡红舌、薄白苔"。

由于舌的一定部位与脏腑相互联系，并反映着相关脏腑的病理变化，所以把舌划分为舌尖、舌中、舌根和舌边（舌的两边）四个部分，分属于心肺、脾胃、肾、肝胆等有关脏腑。

望舌的方法及注意事项：望舌要在充足的自然光线下进行，让患者张口，自然地将舌伸出口外。先看舌苔，并依次观察舌尖、舌中、舌根及舌的两旁，然后再沿舌尖及两旁观察舌质。力求迅速敏捷，必要时，可重复观察 1~2 次。

此外，望舌时应注意"染苔"和其他假象。如乌梅、橄榄等可将舌苔染黑；黄连、黄柏等中药可使舌苔染黄；过热饮食可使舌质变红；刮舌可使舌苔由厚变薄等。因此，在望舌时，除注意伸舌方法、光线外，还需注意其他因素的影响，才能获得正确的观察结果。

1. **望舌质** 望舌质包括观察舌的颜色和形态两方面的异常变化，其侧重于反映脏腑气血的病变。

（1）望舌色：

1）舌色较正常淡，称为淡白舌。主寒证、虚证。多为阳气衰弱、气血不足之象。

2）舌色较正常深，称为红舌。多属热证。

3）舌色深红，称为绛色。多属热盛。

4）舌见紫色，多属瘀血。

（2）望形态：

1）舌体较正常者胖大，为胖大舌。舌淡白而胖，多属脾肾阳虚；舌深红而胖，多属心脾热盛。

2）舌体瘦小而薄，为瘦薄舌，是阴血亏损之象。瘦薄而色淡者，多属心脾两虚、气血不足；瘦薄红绛而干者，是阴虚火旺，病情较重。

3）舌体上有各种形状的裂沟，称裂纹舌。若舌红绛而有裂纹，多为热盛伤阴；舌淡白而有裂纹，多属气血不足。

4）舌体边缘有牙齿的痕迹，称齿痕舌。其多因舌体胖大而受齿缘压迫所致，故齿痕舌常与胖大舌同见。多属脾虚湿盛。

5）舌乳头增生、肥大，高起如刺者，称芒刺舌。多为热邪内结的表现。

2. **望舌苔**　望舌苔包括观察苔质与苔色两方面的异常变化，其侧重反映病邪的深浅、疾病的轻重及发展变化。

（1）望苔色：

1）白苔主表证、寒证。

2）黄苔主热证、里证。黄苔的颜色越深，其热越重。

3）灰苔主里证，可见于里热证，亦可见于寒湿证。

4）黑苔主里证，主热极，又主寒盛。常见于疾病的严重阶段

（2）望苔质：

1）舌苔的润燥，主要是反映津液变化的情况。苔面有过多的水分，称滑苔，多是水湿内盛；苔面干燥，称为燥苔，多为热盛伤津，或阴津不足所致。

2）苔质疏松而厚，如豆腐渣，刮之易去，称为腐苔；若舌面覆盖一层滑黏苔垢，刮之难去，称为腻苔。腐腻苔多见于湿浊、痰饮或食积等病症。

二、闻诊

闻诊，是指通过听声音和嗅气味两个方面，以推断病情的一种诊察方法。听声音，主要是听患者的语言、呼吸及咳嗽等变化；嗅气味，主要是嗅患者的口气、分泌物及排泄物的异常气味。

（一）听声音

1. **听语声**　患者语声的强弱，一方面反映正气的盛衰，同时也与邪气的性质有关。如语声高亢洪亮，多言烦躁者，多属实证、热证；语声低微无力，少言沉静者，多属虚证、寒证。

2. **听呼吸声**　呼吸微弱、短而声低，多属内伤虚损；呼吸有力、声高气粗，多属热邪内盛。呼吸困难、张口抬肩、难于平卧者，称为"喘"。喘有虚实之分，若喘息气粗、声高息涌，属实喘；喘而声低、呼多吸少、气不连续，多属虚喘。

3. **听咳嗽声**　咳声重浊，多属实证；咳声低微气弱，多属虚证。咳痰不爽，痰

稠色黄，多属肺热；咳痰容易，量多色白，多是寒痰或湿痰阻肺；干咳无痰或少量黏痰，多属燥邪犯肺或阴虚肺燥。

（二）嗅气味

口气臭秽，多见于胃热或消化不良，亦见于龋齿、口腔不洁等；口气酸臭，多是胃有宿食；咳吐浊痰脓血，有腥臭味，多属肺痈；鼻流浊涕且臭，多属肺热鼻渊；大便臭秽为热，气腥属寒；小便臊臭混浊，多为湿热下注；矢气酸臭，多为宿食停滞；月经臭秽属热，气腥属寒；带下臭稠，多属湿热；带下气腥，多属虚寒。

三、问诊

医生对患者或其陪诊者进行有目的的询问，这种诊察方法称问诊。患者的一般情况、现病史、既往史、个人史和家族史等，均要通过问诊才能了解。

问诊的目的，在于采集与辨证论治有关的资料，以了解病变的部位、性质、病因、邪正虚实情况。

问诊时，医生的态度要和蔼可亲，语言要通俗简洁，工作要严肃认真，对患者的疾苦要热情关心。只有倾听患者主诉，取得患者的配合，才能得到比较完整准确的病情资料，为诊断治疗提供可靠的依据。

（一）问寒热

疾病初起，恶寒与发热同时并见，多为外感表证；如恶寒重发热轻，多属风寒表证；发热重恶寒轻，多属风热表证。

患者只发热不恶寒，兼口渴便秘，多为里热实证；久病畏寒，不发热或手足发凉，多为阳气虚弱；久病午后或入夜发热，兼颧红、盗汗、五心烦热，多为阴虚内热。

（二）问汗

问汗应问清楚汗的多少，出汗的时间、部位和性质，以辨别其病因为人体内邪气有余，还是为正气不足。

无汗发热恶寒，多为表实证；有汗发热恶风，多为表虚证；汗出量多，兼高热、烦渴，多为里实热证；大汗淋漓、神疲气弱、脉微、肢冷，是阳虚气脱危证。

经常汗出不止，活动时更甚，肢体乏力，称为"自汗"，多属气虚、阳虚；睡后汗出而黏，醒后即止，谓之"盗汗"，多属阴虚。

此外，如先见战栗，继而汗出，称为"战汗"，病势危重；汗出如油、淋漓不止，称"绝汗"。

（三）问痛

痛，是临床上最常见的自觉症状之一。问痛，主要是询问疼痛的部位、性质、程度和时间等。

1. **问头痛** 头痛突然发作，痛势较剧多属实证；经常性头痛，多属虚证；头痛不止，兼恶寒发热，多为外感头痛；时痛时止，每兼眩晕，多为内伤头痛。

2. **问身痛** 身痛兼寒热头痛，多为表证；兼发热口渴，多为里热证。关节疼痛，每逢阴雨或天气变化而加重者，多为"痹证"。痛处游走不定为"行痹"（风痹）；痛有定处，疼痛剧烈为"痛痹"（寒痹）；痛处固定，肢体沉重麻木为"着痹"（湿痹）。

腰痛酸楚而无力，小便清长，多为肾阳虚；腰痛腰酸兼便秘、尿赤，多为肾阴虚；腰部冷痛，如坐水中，似带重物，多为湿邪过盛；腰痛如锥刺，痛处不移，难于转侧，多为血瘀。

3. **问胸腹痛** 胸腹为五脏六腑所居之处，故脏腑出现病变时，常从胸腹反映出来。

胸中冷痛，咳吐痰沫，多为寒邪犯肺；胸中热痛、烦渴者，多为热邪犯肺；胸胁作痛，痛如针刺，多为瘀血；胸痛，咳吐脓血腥臭，多为肺痈；胸痛、潮热、盗汗、干咳少痰或痰中带血，多为肺痨；胸痛彻背，或背痛彻胸，为胸痹。

腹痛隐隐，遇冷加重，或吐涎沫，多为寒证；腹痛拒按，喜冷便秘，多为实证；腹痛喜按喜暖，或便溏，多为虚证；腹部胀痛，嗳腐吞酸，多为食滞；脐周疼痛，时作时止，多为虫积。

（四）问饮食、口味

问饮食、口味的情况，可了解脏腑的虚实和功能盛衰。对脾胃功能盛衰所引起的疾病诊断，本项询问有着尤为重要的意义。

问饮食、口味，主要是询问患者的食欲、食量、口渴、饮水及口味变化等。

1. **问食欲及食量** 病情中食量渐增，多为胃气渐复的表现；食量渐减，多为脾胃虚弱的表现。消谷善饥，多为胃火炽盛；饥而不食，多为胃阴不足。厌食、厌油腻、厌肥甘厚味，多见于肝胆、脾胃湿热内蕴的病症。嗜食异物（生米、泥土等），多见于小儿虫积。妇女妊娠，可有厌食或嗜偏食，一般不属病态。

2. **问口渴与饮水** 口渴多饮且欲饮冷，多属热盛伤津；渴喜热饮，饮量不多，属于中寒或湿盛；大渴引饮，小便反多，多为消渴。

3. **问口味** 口苦，属热，多为肝胆热盛；口甜而黏腻，多为脾胃湿热；口中泛酸，多为肝胃蕴热；口中有酸腐味，多为伤食积滞；口中味咸，多为肾虚；口淡乏味，多为脾虚失运，或水湿内停。

（五）问二便

主要询问大小便的次数、性状、颜色、气味以及有无出血等情况。

1. **问大便** 便秘兼腹满胀痛或发热口渴，多为实证、热证；久病、老人、孕妇或产后便秘，多属津亏血少，或气阴两虚。腹痛即泄，肛门灼热，小便短赤，为热泻；腹冷便溏，腹痛绵绵，不思饮食，为寒泻；长期黎明前腹痛泄泻，称为"五更泻"，属肾阳虚衰；便溏酸臭，腹胀腹痛，里急后重，为湿热痢疾。

2. **问小便** 小便清长而多，多属虚寒；小便短少黄赤，多为热证；若兼尿痛、排尿不畅而混浊，多为膀胱湿热；小便频数，甚至自遗或失禁，多为肾虚或气虚。

（六）问睡眠

问睡眠，可以了解机体阴阳盛衰的情况。如患者失眠、食欲减退、倦怠乏力、心悸健忘、面色无华，多为思虑过度、心脾两虚；虚烦失眠、潮热盗汗、舌红少津，多为阴虚内热；夜眠不安、少睡易醒、口舌生疮，多为心火亢盛；失眠多梦、头痛口苦、急躁易怒，多为肝胆火盛。若患者多睡、肢体困重，多为湿盛；体倦乏力而嗜睡，多为阳气虚弱；食后困倦多睡，多为脾气不足；病后嗜睡，多为正气还未复原之象。

（七）问经带

经、带、胎、产是女性特有的生理现象，一旦产生异常改变常反映出疾病的存在，所以对女性患者，必须详细询问经带情况。

月经先期，色鲜红而量多，多为血热；色淡量少，腹痛喜按，多为气血两虚。月经后期，色紫暗有块，经前腹痛，多为瘀血或寒证；经行无定期，腹痛拒按，或经前乳胀，多为肝郁气滞。

闭经，兼见神疲气短、面色无华，多为血虚；如兼精神抑郁、舌质紫暗，多为血瘀。已婚者，平素体健，忽然停经，呕吐择食、脉滑而匀，多为妊娠。

带下量多稀白，多为脾肾虚寒；量多色黄、质稠臭秽，多为湿热内盛；赤白带下、稠黏臭秽，多为湿毒。

四、切诊

切诊，是医生用手在患者身上的一定部位，进行触、摸、按、压，以了解病情的诊法。它可分为脉诊和按诊两个部分。

（一）脉诊

脉诊，又称"切脉"，是中医诊断学的重要组成部分，医生常通过对脉象的诊断来了解病情，脉诊目前主要运用"寸口诊法"，寸口脉分为寸、关、尺三部，即掌后桡动脉浅表部位。具体来说：掌后高骨（桡骨茎突）的部位为"关"，关前（腕端）为"寸"，关后（肘端）为"尺"。医生用自己的食指、中指及无名指分别放在寸、关、尺部位，两手寸、关、尺共为六部。左手寸关尺分别对应的脏腑为心、肝胆、肾；右手寸关尺分别对应的脏腑为肺、脾胃、命门。

诊脉时，应先让患者稍事休息，然后令其平坐或仰卧，手臂平伸与心位置齐高，掌心向上平放（仰掌式），或要患者伸手曲肘，前臂和掌心侧置（曲肘式）。医者先以中指对准高骨（桡骨茎突），再用食指按关前的寸部，无名指按在关后的尺部。布指的疏密，可视患者身材的高矮而定。

按脉时，医生要呼吸均匀，心平气和，集中注意力，以自己的自然呼吸（一呼一吸为一息）次数或钟表计时来计算患者的脉搏至数，细心体察脉搏的浅深部位、次数快慢等变化，以判断疾病的情况。

（二）按诊

按诊，是对患者的肌肤、手足、腹部及病变部位进行触摸按压，以探察局部温凉、软硬、压痛及痞块等情况，从而推断疾病部位和性质的一种诊察方法。

1. **按肌表**　主要辨别肌肤体表的寒热、润燥、肿胀及疼痛等。

2. **按手足**　主要是了解手足的寒热。

3. **按腹部**　主要是了解脘腹的疼痛、软硬以及有无结节硬块等异物的情况。

第二章　养生适宜技术基础操作

第一节　针刺法

针刺法是采用适当的针具在人体上刺激一定的穴位来激发机体的抗病能力，调整机体阴阳、气血、脏腑，以达到防病目的的一种治疗方法。临床上常用的有毫针法、水针法、耳针法、皮内针法和电针法等。本书重点介绍一下毫针刺法的操作规范。

毫针刺法是临床上应用广泛的一种方法。

1 适应范围　各种急、慢性疾病，如中风、偏头疼、三叉神经痛、坐骨神经痛、膈肌痉挛、痛经、荨麻疹、颈椎病、急性腰扭伤、腰肌劳损、牙痛等。

2. 禁忌证

1）患者疲乏、饥饿或精神高度紧张时。

2）皮肤有感染、瘢痕或肿痛部位时。

3）有出血倾向及高度水肿时。

4）小儿囟门未闭合及头顶腧穴不宜针刺。

3. 物品准备　2%碘酊、75%酒精（乙醇）、无菌棉签、棉球、镊子、毫针盒清洁弯盘，必要时备毛毯或浴巾、垫枕、屏风等。

4. 操作方法

（1）进针法：

1）指切进针法，又称爪切进针法。用左手拇指或食指端按腧穴位置旁边，右手持针紧靠左手指甲面将针刺入腧穴。此法适宜于短针的进针，如内关、照海等穴。

2）夹持进针法或称骈指进针法。即用左手拇、食二指捏消毒干棉球，夹住针身下端，将针尖固定在所刺入腧穴皮肤表面位置，右手捻动针柄，将针刺入腧穴。

此法适用于肌肉丰满部位腧穴及长针的进针，如环跳、秩边等穴。

3）舒张进针法是用左手拇、食二指将所刺腧穴部位的皮肤绷紧，右手持针。使针从左手拇、食二指的中间刺入。此法主要指用于皮肤松弛或有皱折的部位的腧穴，如腹部的关元、天枢等穴。

4）提捏进针法是用左手拇、食二指将所刺腧穴部位的皮肤捏紧，右手持针，从捏起的皮肤顶端将针刺入。此法主要用于皮肉浅薄部位的腧穴进针，如印堂、攒竹等穴。

（2）进针的角度和深度：

1）针刺的角度，是指进针时针身与皮肤表面所构成的夹角，一般常见的针刺角度有直刺、斜刺和平刺三种。

直刺：是针身与皮肤表面呈90°角左右垂直刺入。此法适用于人体大部分腧穴。

斜刺：是针身与皮肤表面呈45°角左右倾斜刺入。此法适用于肌肉较浅薄处、内有重要脏器处或不宜于直刺、深刺的腧穴。

平刺：即沿皮刺，是针身与皮肤表面呈15°～25°角沿皮刺入。此法适用于皮薄肉少部位的腧穴。

2）针刺的深度，是指针身刺入皮肉的深浅，其把握原则是既要获得针感又不伤及重要脏器。

体质：身体瘦弱者，宜浅刺；身强体肥者，宜深刺。

年龄：年老体弱及小儿娇嫩之体，宜浅刺；中青年身强体壮者，宜深刺。

病情：阳证、新病者宜浅刺；阴证、久病者，宜深刺。

部位：头面和胸背及皮薄肉少处的腧穴，宜浅刺；四肢、臀部、腹部及肌肉丰满处的腧穴，宜深刺。

（3）行针基本手法：

1）提插法是当针刺入腧穴一定深度后，将针身提到浅层，再由浅层插到深层，以加大刺激量，使局部产生酸、麻、胀、重等感觉。

2）捻转法是指当针刺入腧穴的一定深度后，将针身大幅度一前一后交替捻转，幅度愈大，频率愈快，刺激量也就愈大。当针刺部位出现酸麻、胀、重等感觉时，术者手下也会有沉、紧、涩的感觉，即为"得气"，说明针刺起到了作用。

（4）补泻手法：　一般轻刺激为补，重刺激为泻，中等刺激为平补平泻。虚证多用补法，实证多用泻法。

1）补法。进针慢而浅，提插轻，捻转幅度小，留针后不捻转，出针后多揉按针孔。多用于虚证。

2）泻法。进针快而深，提插重，捻转幅度大，留针时间长，并反复捻转，出针时不按针孔。多用于实证。

3）平补平泻。进针深浅适中，刺激强度适宜，提插和捻转的幅度中等，进针和出针用力均匀。适用于一般患者。

5. 操作步骤

1）备齐物品，携至床旁，核对姓名、诊断及处方腧穴，并请患者排空小便。

2）对初次接受针刺治疗的患者，介绍有关情况（如酸、胀、麻、重等针感以及各种副反应出现的可能），以解除患者的恐惧心理。

3）按腧穴不同取适当体位，协助患者松开衣物。并用大小不同的垫子垫好，使患者采取平衡舒适而能持久的姿势。

4）选好腧穴后，先用拇指按压穴位，并询问患者的感觉反应。

5）用 2% 碘酊消毒进针部位后，按腧穴深浅和患者胖瘦，选取合适的毫针，同时检查针柄是否松动，针身和针尖是否弯曲或带钩。术者用 75% 酒精棉球消毒手指后，再用 75% 酒精棉球局部脱碘。

6）进针。左手拇（食）指端切按在腧穴旁边，右手持针，用拇、食、中三指挟持针柄近针根处，将针尖对准腧穴迅速刺入皮肤，缓慢捻转进针。此法多用于 1.5 寸以内的毫针（若用 3 寸以上长毫针时，可采用夹持进针法，即左手拇、食指捏消毒干棉球夹住针身下端，将针尖固定在所刺腧穴皮肤表面，右手拇、食、中三指夹持针柄，快速将针刺入皮肤，同时右手配合下压，并将针捻转进入深处）。

7）当刺入一定深度时患者产生局部酸、麻、胀、重等感觉，或向远处扩散，即为"得气"。得气后按病情需要运用补泻手法调节针感或适当留针，一般留针 10 ～ 20 分钟。

8）在针刺及留针过程中，密切观察有无晕针、滞针、弯针、折针或气胸等情况。随时准备相应的处理。

9）起针。左手拇（食）指端按压在针孔周围皮肤处，右手持针柄慢慢捻动将针尖退至皮下，迅速将针拔出，随即用无菌干棉球轻轻按压针孔片刻，防止出血。最后检查起针数目，以防遗漏。

10）操作完毕，协助患者穿好衣裤，安置适宜卧位，整理床单，清理用物，归还原处，洗手。

11）记录操作过程、腧穴、留针时间、反应及效果等，要求患者签名。

6. 针刺意外的处理及预防

（1）晕针：进针后患者出现头晕、目眩、面色苍白、胸闷欲呕、出汗肢冷、心慌气短等晕厥现象，称为晕针。

1）处理。立即出针，使患者去枕平卧，给饮热水或糖水，闭目休息片刻，即可恢复。重症可指掐或针刺人中、足三里、内关，灸百会、气海等穴，休息片刻即可恢复。

2）预防。①对初诊体弱、老年人、血管神经机能不稳定、饥饿过劳及康复期患者，应取卧位针刺，手法宜轻。②诊室内注意通风，冬季注意保暖。③随时观察患者反应，以便及早发现晕针先兆，及时处理。

（2）出血及血肿：多因刺伤血管，起针时没有及时按压所致。

1）处理。①点状出血可用无菌干棉球按压针孔。②青紫块或血肿，早期可压迫止血或冷敷，晚期可进行热敷。③头部血肿者，可在无菌操作下穿刺抽血，继续加压包扎。

2）预防。①熟悉腧穴、经络位置，以免刺伤血管。②有出血倾向者，忌用针刺。

（3）弯针：指针身在患者体内发生弯曲的现象。

1）处理。若发生弯针，不宜再运针。若因体位改变引起，应先矫正体位再起针。若弯曲的角度较大，可以轻轻摇动针体，顺着弯曲的方向慢慢退出。

2）预防。手法指力须均匀，刺激不宜突然加大，体位要舒适，指导患者勿随意更动体位，防止外物碰撞和压迫。

（4）滞针：是指因患者精神紧张，针刺入后，局部肌肉强烈收缩，或刺入肌腱，或行针时单向捻转致肌纤维缠绕针身，使针在体内一时性的捻转不动，而且有进退不得的现象。

1）处理。①对惧针者，应耐心安慰，并嘱患者进行深呼吸，待肌肉松弛后再起针。②轻弹针柄或按摩穴位四周或在滞针附近再刺1～2针，以解肌肉痉挛，然后起针。③对因肌纤维缠绕者，可向反方向捻转，待肌纤维回解后再起针。

2）预防。对初诊患者应做好解释工作。操作时捻针幅度不宜过大。平时检查针具时，对不符合质量要求的针具应剔出不用。

（5）折针：指针在体内发生折断，残端留在体内的现象。

1）处理。①发现折针，应嘱患者不要移动体位，以防断针向深处陷入。②如折断处尚有部分露出皮肤外，可用止血钳取出；若未露出皮肤表面，可用手按压周围皮肤，使残端露出皮肤外，再用止血钳取出。③若用以上方法取针无效，应采用外科手术取出。

2）预防。①针刺及留针过程中，切勿将针身全部刺入（要求留出针身1/4以上）。②针具须定期按标准检查，凡质量不合要求者，应弃去不用。③捻针时，忌用强力。若发生滞针及弯针时，处理要得当，以防折针。

（6）气胸：指针刺胸背部穴位过深，误伤肺脏，空气进入胸腔，引起外伤性气胸。

1）处理。①一旦发现气胸，应立即报告医生，并让患者取半坐卧位休息。严密观察病情变化。②避免咳嗽。必要时遵医嘱给予抗感染治疗。③重病者应积极配合医生行胸腔穿刺减压术。

2）预防。①凡在胸、背锁骨上窝及胸骨上窝部穴位进行针刺治疗时，应严格掌握进针的角度和深度。②对哮喘、老年性慢性支气管炎、肺气肿患者，在上述各部位针刺时，更应谨慎。

第二节　灸法

灸法是以艾绒为主要原料，制成艾条或艾炷，点燃后在人体某穴位或患处熏灸的一种治疗方法。利用温热及药物的作用，通过经络传导，以温通经络、调和气血、消肿散结、祛湿散寒、回阳救逆，从而达到防病保健、治病强身的目的。

一、艾条灸

用纯净的艾绒（或加入中药）卷成圆柱形的艾卷，点燃后在人体表面熏灸的一种技术操作。

1.适应范围　痹病、脾虚、宫寒、中风、脱证、胎位不正等，亦可用于防病保健。

2.禁忌证

1）实热证、阴虚发热者不宜施灸。

2）颜面部、大血管处。

3）不宜施灸。孕妇腹部及腰骶部不宜施灸。

3. **物品准备**　治疗盘、艾条、点火用具、弯盘、小口瓶，必要时备浴巾、屏风等。

4. **操作方法**

1）备齐物品携至床旁，做好解释，再次核对。

2）取合理体位，暴露施灸部位，冬季注意保暖。

3）根据病情或医嘱，实施相应的灸法。

温和灸：点燃艾条，将点燃的一端，在距离施灸穴位皮肤3厘米左右处进行熏灸，以局部有温热感而无灼痛为宜。一般每处灸5～7分钟，至局部皮肤红晕为度。

雀啄灸：将艾条点燃的一端，在距离施灸部位2～5厘米，如同鸟雀啄食般，一上一下不停地移动，反复熏灸，每处5分钟左右。

回旋灸：将艾条点燃的一端，距施灸部位3厘米左右，来回旋转移动，进行反复熏灸，一般可灸20～30分钟。

5. **注意事项**

1）施灸部位，宜先上后下，先灸头顶、胸背，后灸腹部、四肢。

2）施灸过程中，随时询问患者有无灼痛感，及时调节距离，防止烧伤。观察病情变化及有无因体位不适引起的机体痛苦，了解患者的生理、心理感受。

3）施灸中应及时将艾灰弹入弯盘，防止烧伤皮肤及烧坏衣物。

4）施灸完毕，立即将艾条插入小口瓶。熄灭艾火。清洁患者局部皮肤后，协助患者穿好衣着，安置舒适卧位，酌情开窗通风。

5）清理用物，归还原处，洗手，记录并签名。

6）施灸后局部皮肤出现微红灼热，属于正常现象。如灸后出现小水疱，无须处理，可自行吸收。如水疱较大，可用无菌注射器抽去水疱内液体，覆盖消毒纱布，保持干燥，防止感染。

二、艾炷灸

艾炷灸是将纯净的艾绒搓捏成圆锥状（如麦粒大或如半截枣核，大小不等），直接或间接置于穴位上施灸的一种技术操作。分为直接灸和间接灸两种。

1. **适应范围**　参照本章第二节"艾条灸"部分。

2. **禁忌证**　参照本章第二节"艾条灸"部分。

3. **物品准备** 治疗盘、艾炷、点火用具、凡士林、棉签、镊子、弯盘，酌情备浴巾、屏风等。间接灸时，备姜片或蒜片等。

4. **操作方法**

1）备齐物品，携至床旁，做好解释，核对医嘱。

2）取合理体位，暴露施灸部位，注意保暖。

3）根据医嘱实施相应的灸法。

直接灸（常用无瘢痕灸）：先在施灸部位涂以少量凡士林，放置艾炷后点燃，艾炷燃烧至 2/5 左右，或患者感到灼痛时，即用镊子取走余下的艾炷，放于弯盘中，更换新炷再灸，一般连续灸 5 ～ 7 壮。

间接灸（常用隔姜灸、隔蒜灸、隔盐灸或隔附子饼灸）：施灸部位涂凡士林，根据医嘱，放上鲜姜片或蒜片或附子饼 1 片（先将鲜姜或独头蒜切成约 0.6 厘米厚的薄片，中心处用针穿刺数孔；附子饼是附子研末以黄酒调和而成，厚 0.6 ～ 0.9 厘米，中心用粗针穿数孔），上置艾炷，点燃施灸。当艾炷燃尽或患者感到灼痛时，则更换新炷再灸，一般灸 3 ～ 7 壮。达到灸处皮肤出现红晕，不起水疱为度。

5. **注意事项**

1）施灸部位，宜先上后下，先灸头顶、胸背，后灸腹部、四肢。

2）采用艾炷时，针柄上的艾绒必须捻紧，防止艾灰脱落烧伤皮肤，或烧坏衣物。

3）艾炷燃烧时，应认真观察，防止艾灰脱落，以免灼伤皮肤或烧坏衣物等。

4）熄灭后的艾炷，应装入小口瓶内，以防复燃，发生火灾。

5）施灸完毕，清洁局部皮肤，协助患者衣着。整理床单，安排舒适体位，酌情开窗通风。

6）清理用物，归还原处。洗手，记录并签名。

7）施灸后局部皮肤出现微红灼热，属于正常现象。如灸后出现小水疱，无须处理，可自行吸收。如水疱较大，可用无菌注射器抽去水疱内液体，覆盖消毒纱布，保持干燥，防止感染。

第三节 拔罐疗法

拔罐疗法又称为"火罐法""吸筒法"，是指运用各种罐具，经过排除其中的空气产生负压，使之吸附于皮肤表面，通过局部的负压和温热作用，引起局部组织充血和皮内轻微的瘀血，促使该处的经络通畅，气血旺盛，以刺激经络腧穴或拔毒排脓，从而达到相应治疗作用的一种常用的外治方法。具有活血、行气、止痛、消肿、散结、退热、祛风、散寒、除湿、拔毒等作用，广泛地运用于内、外、妇、儿、骨伤、皮肤、五官等科症病的治疗。

1. 适应范围

1）风湿痹痛及各种神经麻痹。

2）感冒、痰饮、咳喘。

3）胃脘痛、腹痛、腰背痛、脚气病。

4）痈疽疮疡初起未溃。

2. 禁忌证

1）急性危重疾病、严重心脏病、心力衰竭患者。

2）皮肤高度过敏者，接触性传染病以及皮肤肿瘤（肿块）部位，皮肤溃烂部位。

3）血小板减少性紫癜、血友病等凝血功能异常疾病患者。

4）心尖区、体表动脉搏动处及静脉曲张处。

5）精神分裂症、抽搐、高度紧张及不合作者。

6）急性外伤性骨折部位，中度和重度水肿部位。

7）瘰疬、疝气处及活动性肺结核患者。

8）眼、耳、口、鼻等五官孔窍处。

9）佩戴心脏起搏器等精密金属植入物的受术者，禁用电罐、磁罐。

10）醉酒者、过于消瘦者、过度疲劳者。

3. 物品准备

（1）施术前准备：

1）罐具。根据操作部位、操作方法的不同选择相应的罐具。将罐具对准光源以确定罐体完整无裂痕，用手触摸以确定罐口内外光滑无毛糙。对罐具消毒，其内壁应擦拭干净。常用罐的种类玻璃罐、竹罐及其他罐具等。

2）部位。应根据治未病目的选取适当的操作部位。常用部位为具有保健及防治疾病作用的相关腧穴以及肌肉丰厚处。

（2）体位：应选择受术者舒适且能持久保持的、便于施术者操作的体位。

（3）术前准备及注意事项：应保持全身肌肉放松，并做好充足的心理准备。

施术者应注意观察受术者状态，如有紧张、恐惧、焦虑或肌肉紧张等情况出现，应做心理减压辅导，严重者应及时终止操作。

（4）环境：保持环境清洁卫生，避免污染，环境温度应保持26℃左右。

（5）消毒：

1）罐具消毒。对不同材质、用途的罐具可用不同的消毒方法。

2）施术部位消毒。一般拔罐的部位不需要消毒，应保持施术部位皮肤清洁。应用针罐法、刺络放血法时使用75%酒精或0.5%～1%聚维酮碘（碘伏）棉球在施术部位消毒。

3）施术者消毒。施术者双手可用肥皂水清洗干净，应用针罐法、刺络拔罐法时再用75%酒精棉球擦拭。

4.操作方法

（1）火罐法：利用燃烧时火焰的热力，排出空气，形成负压，将罐吸拔在皮肤上。它是最常用的一种方法，一般疾病均可采用。

（2）蒸汽罐法：用竹罐置水内煮沸，使用时用镊子将罐子夹出，甩去水液，迅速按拔在皮肤上，即可吸住。

（3）抽气罐法：将罐贴紧皮肤，用抽气枪将罐中的空气抽出，产生负压，即将罐吸住。

（4）水气罐法：按抽气罐法操作将罐吸拔于皮肤上后，注入3毫升左右生理盐水或蒸馏水，以保持罐内皮肤湿润，以防因负压过高而造成皮肤渗血。

（5）煮药拔罐法：把配制成的药物装入袋内，放入水中煮至适当浓度，再将竹罐投入药汁内煮10～15分钟。使用时按蒸汽罐法吸拔于患处。此法多用于风湿类病。

（6）贮药罐：其操作方法有两种，一种是抽气罐内事先盛贮一定量的药液，约为罐子的1/2，快速紧扣于被拔部位，然后按抽气罐法，抽出罐内空气，即可吸拔于皮肤上。另一种是在玻璃火罐内盛贮一定的药液，约为罐子的1/2，然后按火罐法快速吸拔在皮肤上。

（7）针罐法：先在穴位上针刺，待施毕补泻手法后，将针留在原处，再以针刺为中心拔上火罐即可。如果与药罐结合，称为针药罐法。此法不宜使用过长过细的针，留在体外的针身、针柄不宜过长。此法多用于风湿痹痛。

5. 操作步骤

1）仔细检查患者，明确临床诊断，根据病情决定拔罐方法。

2）需应用的药品、器材齐备，并一一擦净，按次序排列好。

3）施术。首先将选好的部位显露出来，术前靠近患者身边，顺手（或左或右手）执罐按不同方法扣上。一般有两种排序：

密排法：罐与罐之间的距离不超过3厘米，用于身体强壮且有疼痛症状者。有镇静、止痛、消炎之功。又称"刺激法"。

疏排法：罐与罐之间的距离相隔3～6厘米。用于身体衰弱、肢体麻木、酸软无力者。又称"弱刺激法"。

4）询问。火罐拔上后，应频繁询问患者有感觉（假如用玻璃罐，还要观察罐内皮肤反应情况），如果罐吸力过大，产生疼痛即应放入少量空气。方法是左手拿住罐体稍倾斜，以右手指按压对侧的皮肤，使之形成一个微小的空隙，让空气徐徐进入，入气适度时即应停止，重新扣好。拔罐后患者如感到吸着无力，可起下来再拔一次。如有其他情况，则应予以对症处理。

5）留罐时间。大罐吸力强，每次可拔5～10分钟；小罐吸力弱，每次可拔10～15分钟。此外还应根据患者的年龄、体质、病情、病程，以及拔罐的施术部位而灵活掌握。

6）拔罐次数。每日或隔日1次，一般10次为1个疗程，中间休息3～5日。特殊的罐法依具体情况而定。

7）起罐。用一只手拿住罐子，另一只手按罐口边的皮肤，两手协作，待空气缓缓进入罐内后（空气进入太快则负压骤减容易使患者产生疼痛），罐即落下，切不可用力起拔，以免损伤皮肤。

8）起罐后处理。一般不需进行处理。如留罐时间过长，皮肤起较大的水疱时，可用消毒针刺破后，涂以甲紫溶液，以防感染。拔罐后如针孔出血，则可用干的消毒棉球压迫止血。如局部出血严重，再次拔罐时应避开此处。处理完毕后，让患者休息10～20分钟后方可离去。

6. 注意事项

1）选择肌肉丰满，毛发少的部位拔罐。肌肉瘦削、骨骼凹凸不平及毛发多部位不能应用。

2）根据病情和不同部位，采用不同的拔罐方法，选用大小合适口径的罐（或瓶）。患者体位要舒适。

3）操作时谨防烫伤皮肤。点火入罐时动作要敏捷，避免烫伤皮肤，或先于局部涂以凡士林，既能增强吸着力，又能防罐口灼伤皮肤。在点火过程中如发现罐口发烫，应当换罐；应用闪火法和滴酒法时，防止燃着的棉花掉下；应用架火法时，不要将点燃的火架撞翻；应用蒸汽罐和煮药罐时，应甩去罐中的热水和药液，以防引起烫伤。

4）在应用针罐时，避免将针撞压入深处，防止弯针和折针。

5）在应用刺血拔罐时，刺血工具要严格消毒，出血量要适当。眼区及面颊部不宜采用。体质虚弱、贫血、肿瘤患者、出血性疾患，孕妇、月经期不宜采用此法治疗。

6）在应用走罐时，罐口应光滑，不宜吸拔过紧，不能在骨突出处推拉，以免损伤皮肤。

7）留罐时间不宜太久以免皮肤起疱，引起烫伤，一般以 10 分钟为宜。如烫伤时，可涂甲紫溶液或烫伤膏即可，并防止感染。

8）起罐时手法宜轻缓，以一手抵住罐口边的肌肉，按压一下，使空气透入，罐子即能脱下，不可硬行单向上提或旋转。

9）拔罐后如局部瘀血严重或者疼痛时，轻轻按摩被拔部位即可缓解，在局部瘀血现象尚未消退以前，不宜再在此处拔罐。

10）患者如有晕罐现象，应立即起罐，及时做妥善处理。

7. 拔罐的反应及处理

（1）反应：

1）正常反应。不论采用何种方法将罐吸附于施治部位由于罐内的负压吸拔作用，局部的组织可隆起于罐口平面以上，患者觉得局部有牵拉发胀感，或感到发热、发紧、凉气外出、温暖、舒适等，这都是正常现象。起罐后，或应用闪罐、走罐后，治疗部位出现潮红（或紫红）皮疹点等，均属拔罐疗法的罐后治疗效应，待1 至数天后，可自行恢复，不需做任何处理。

2）异常反应。拔罐后如果患者感到拔罐区异常紧而痛，或有烧灼感受，则应立即拿掉火罐，并检查皮肤有无烫伤，患者是否过度紧张，术者手法是否有误，或罐子吸力是否过大等，根据具体情况予以处理。如此处不宜再行拔罐，可另选其他部位。针后拔罐或刺络（刺血）拔罐时，如罐内有大量出血（超过治疗要求的出血量），应立即起罐，并用消毒棉球按住出血点。

（2）晕罐：晕罐是拔罐治疗中产生的种特殊情况，与晕针有相似之处，常于行罐中发生，起罐后发作，虽不多见，但不可不防。

1）晕罐之症状。头晕目眩，面色苍白，恶心欲吐，呼吸急促，心慌心悸，四肢发凉，伴有冷汗，脉沈细、血压下降；严重者，口唇、指甲青紫，神志昏迷，仆倒在地，二便失禁，脉微细弱欲绝。

2）晕罐之原因。空腹或过度疲劳、剧吐、大汗之后；心情过于紧张；体质虚弱；手法过重，刺激量大，时间过长，皆可晕罐，甚至形成脱证、闭证。

3）晕罐之处理。要患者平卧，注意保暖。轻者服温开水或糖水即可迅速缓和并恢复正常；重者则应弄清是脱证还是闭证。脱证则施温灸以固脱回阳，取百会、中极、关元、气海、涌泉，或隔盐灸神阙穴即可恢复；脉细弱欲脱者，应立即采取其他急救措施。

4）晕罐之预防。术者应注意观察和询问，若大饥大渴，应令进食，稍休息后再做治疗；神情紧张者应做解释，消除顾虑，不可勉强，手法宜轻；术中一旦发现患者出现不适，应立即处理，防患于未然。

第四节　刮痧疗法

刮痧法是应用边缘钝滑的器具，如牛角刮板、瓷匙等物，在患者体表一定部位反复刮动，使局部皮下出现瘀斑的一种治疗方法。此法可使脏腑秽浊之气通达于外，促使周身气血通畅，逐邪外出，从而达到防病治病的目的。

1. 适应证

1）疼痛性疾病、骨关节退行性疾病如颈椎病等。

2）感冒发热、咳嗽等呼吸系统疾病。

3）亚健康、慢性疲劳综合征的防治。

4）痤疮、黄褐斑等损容性疾病。

2. 禁忌证

1）有出血倾向者，如血友病、血小板减少性紫癜、咯血，以及白血病患者等。

2）高度神经质、狂躁不安不合作者。

3）因全身发热引起的头痛、头目昏重抽搐、痉挛患者。

4）中度或重度心脏病、心力衰竭者。

5）急性外伤性骨折部位，全身高度浮肿者（水肿病）。

6）孕妇腰腹部，妇女月经期。

7）皮肤高度过敏者；各种皮肤病及溃疡；施术部位皮肤破损溃烂者；外伤骨折者；或有静脉曲张、癌肿、恶病质、皮肤丧失弹性者。

8）大血管附近、浅显动脉分布处及疤痕处。

9）醉酒者、过于消瘦者、过度疲劳者。

3.**物品准备** 治疗盘，刮具（牛角刮板、瓷匙等），治疗碗内盛少量清水或药液，必要时备浴巾、屏风等。

4.**操作程序**

1）备齐用物携至床旁，做好解释，再次核对。

2）协助患者取合理体位暴露刮痧部位，冬季注意保暖。

3）根据病情或医嘱，确定刮痧部位，常用的部位有头颅部，背部，胸部及四肢。

4）检查刮具边缘是否光滑，有无缺损，以免划刮皮肤。

5）手持刮具，蘸水或药液，在选定的部位，从上至下刮擦皮肤，要向单一方向，不要来回刮。用力要均匀，禁用暴力。

6）如刮背部，应在脊椎两侧沿肋间隙呈弧线由内向外刮，每次刮 8～10 条，每条长 6～15 厘米。

7）刮动数次后，当刮具干涩时，需及时蘸湿再刮，直至皮下呈现红色或紫红色，一般每一部位刮 20 次左右。

8）刮治过程中，随时询问患者有无不适，观察病情及局部皮肤颜色变化，及时调节手法力度。

9）刮痧完毕，清洁局部皮肤后，协助患者着衣，安置舒适卧位。

10）清理用物，归还原处，洗手，记录。

5.**注意事项**

1）室内空气流通，忌对流风，以防复感风寒而加重病情。

2）操作中用力要均匀，勿伤损皮肤。

3）刮痧过程中要随时观察病情变化，发现异常，应立即停刮，并报告医师，配合处理。

4）刮痧后嘱患者保持情绪舒畅，饮食清淡，忌生冷油腻之品。

5）使用过的刮具应消毒后存放备用。

第五节　推拿法

推拿是通过手法作用于人体体表的特定部位，以调节机体的生理、病理状况，达到治病防病目的。

1. 适应范围　各种急、慢性疾病，如腰椎间盘突出症、颈椎病、肩周炎、落枕、急性腰扭伤、慢性腰肌劳损、胃脘痛、慢性腹泻、便秘、偏瘫、小儿腹泻、牙痛等。

2. 禁忌证

1）各种出血性疾病。

2）妇女月经期。

3）孕妇腰腹部。

4）皮肤破损、瘢痕、水肿等部位。

3. 物品准备　治疗盘、治疗巾、浴巾、屏风。

4. 操作步骤

1）向患者说明推拿的作用、方法，以取得合作。

2）检查患者，明确诊断，根据病情决定推拿手法、部位。

3）进行腰腹部按摩时，嘱患者先排尿。

4）患者采取合理舒适体位，必要时协助松开衣物。冬季注意保暖。

5）根据患者的症状、发病部位、年龄及耐受性，选用适宜的手法和刺激强度，进行按摩。

6）操作过程中要随时观察患者对手法的反应，若有不适，应及时调整手法或停止操作，以防发生意外。

7）操作后协助患者整理衣着，安排舒适卧位。

8）洗手，必要时记录。

5. 按摩基本手法　按摩又称推拿。临床中的推拿手法很多，下面仅介绍几种常用手法。

（1）推法：用指、掌或肘部着力于一定部位上，进行单方向的直线按摩。用指称指推法，用掌称掌推法，用肘称肘推法。操作时指、掌、肘要紧贴体表，用力要稳，速度缓慢而均匀，以能使肌肤深层透热而不擦伤皮肤为度。

此法可在人体各部位使用。能提高肌肉的兴奋性，促进血液循环，并有舒筋活络的作用。

（2）"一指禅"推法：用拇指指腹或指端着力于推拿部位，腕部放松，沉肩、垂肘、悬腕，以肘部为支点，前臂做主动摆动，带动腕部摆动和拇指关节做屈伸活动。手法频率每分钟120～160次，压力、频率、摆动幅度要均匀，动作要灵活，操作时要求达到患者有透热感。

常用于头面、胸腹及四肢等处。

（3）揉法：用手掌大鱼际、掌根或拇指指腹着力，腕关节或掌指做轻揉缓和的摆动。操作时压力要轻柔，动作要协调而有节律，一般速度每分钟120～160次。适用于全身各部位。

（4）摩法：用手掌掌面或手指指腹附着于一定部位或穴位，以腕关节连同前臂做节律性的旋转运动。此法操作时肘关节自然弯曲，腕部放松，指掌自然伸直，动作要缓和而协调，频率每分钟120次左右。

（5）擦法（平推法）：用手掌大鱼际、掌根或小鱼际附着在一定部位，进行直线来回摩擦。操作时手指自然伸开，整个指掌要贴在患者体表治疗部位，以肩关节为支点，上臂主动带动手掌做前后或上下往返移动。动作要均匀连续，推动幅度要大，呼吸自然，不可进气，频率每分钟100～120次。此法用于胸腹、肩背、腰臀部及四肢。

（6）搓法：用双手掌面夹住一定部位，相对用力做快速搓揉，同时做上下往返移动。操作时双手要用力对称，搓动要快，移动要慢；手法由轻到重，再由重到轻，由慢到快，再由快到慢。适用于腰背、胁肋及四肢部位，一般作为推拿结束时手法。具有调和气血、舒筋通络的作用。

（7）抹法：用单手或双手拇指指腹紧贴皮肤，做到上下或左右往返移动。操作时用力要轻而不浮，重而不滞。本法适用于头面及颈项部。有开窍镇静、醒脑明目等作用。

（8）振法：用手指端或手掌着力于体表，前臂和手部肌肉静止性强劲地用力，产生振颤动作，操作时力量要集中在指端或手掌上，振动的频率较高，着力较重。此法多用单手操作，也可双手同时进行。适用于全身各部位和穴位。具有祛痰消积、和气理气的作用。

（9）按法：用拇指端、指腹、单掌或双掌（双掌重叠）按压体表，并稍留片刻。操作时着力部位要紧贴体表，不可移动，用力要由轻到重，不可用暴力猛然按压。指按法适用于全身各部穴位；掌按法适用于腰背及腹部。具有放松肌肉、活血止痛的作用。

（10）捏法：用拇指与食指、中指或拇指与其余四指将患处皮肤、肌肉、肌腱捏起，相对用于挤压。操作时要连续向前提捏推行，均匀而有节律。此法适用于头部、颈项部、肩背及四肢。具有舒经活络、行气活血的作用。

（11）拿法：捏而提起谓之拿，即用拇指与食、中两指或拇指与其余四指相对用力，在一定部位或穴位上进行节律性的提捏。操作时用力要由轻而重，不可突然用力，动作要缓和而有连贯性。临床常配合其他手法适用于颈项、肩部及四肢等部位。具有祛风散寒、舒筋通络的作用。

（12）弹法：用一手指指腹紧压住另一手指指甲，受压手指端用力弹出，连续弹击治疗部位。操作时弹击要均匀，频率为每分钟 120 ～ 160 次。此法可用于全身各部，尤以头面、颈项部最为常用。具有舒筋活络、祛风散寒的作用。

（13）掐法：用拇指指甲重刺穴位。掐法是强刺激手法之一，操作时要逐渐用力，达深透为止，不要掐破皮肤。掐后轻揉皮肤，以缓解不适。此法多用于急救和止痛，常掐合谷、人中、足三里等穴。具有疏通血脉、温通经络的作用。

6. 注意事项

1）操作前应修剪指甲，以防损伤患者皮肤。

2）操作时用力要均匀、柔和、有力、持久，禁用暴力。

3）各种出血性疾病、妇女月经期；孕妇腰骶部、腹部以及皮肤破损处、瘢痕等部位，禁用此法。

第六节　埋线疗法

埋线疗法是在中医的脏腑、气血、经络理论指导下，把羊肠线或生物蛋白线埋植在相应腧穴和特定部位，利用其对穴位的持续刺激作用来治疗疾病。

1. 适应证及疗程　埋线疗法多用于治疗慢性疾病，应该根据疾病的特点、病情选择适当的穴位。治疗间隔及疗程根据病情以及所选部位对线的吸收程度而定，间隔时间 1 周至 1 个月 1 次，视病情 3 ～ 5 次为一个疗程。

2. 禁忌证

1）有出血倾向、精神紧张、大汗、劳累后或饥饿时慎用埋线疗法。

2）埋线时应根据不同穴位选择适当的深度和角度，埋线的部位不应妨碍机体的正常功能和活动，关节、颜面部位及疤痕体质者禁止埋线。

3）有皮肤病、炎症、溃疡、破损处疤痕组织处禁止埋线。

4）糖尿病、蛋白质过敏者及其他各种疾病导致皮肤和皮下组织吸收和修复功能障碍者禁止埋线。

5）孕妇的下腹部和腰骶部及妇女月经期禁止埋线。

3. 物品准备

1）线体选择。可吸收性外科缝线（长度 0.5 ～ 1.0 厘米）。

2）一次性使用埋线针（0.7 毫米 ×55 毫米）。

3）埋线包（包括剪刀、治疗盘、镊子）。

4）无菌手套、口罩、帽子、皮肤消毒剂、棉签、无菌敷料贴。

4. 操作前准备

（1）可吸收性外科缝线处理：开包后即剪即用，长度 1 厘米左右。

（2）穴位选择：根据患者病情选取穴位，穴位应选择肌肉丰富部位，常用腹部、腰背部，慎用头面部穴位如风池等，禁用关节腔、关节、踝、腕关节以下穴位以及血管、神经干分布部位穴位（如内关、三阴交等），穴位数量控制在 ≤ 20 个。

（3）体位选择：根据取穴情况选择不同卧位。

（4）环境要求：操作房间清洁卫生，空气消毒。

（5）消毒：

1）术者及助手手部消毒：双手应进行外科手术消毒规范消毒。

2）器械消毒：埋线包消毒要求达到国家规定的医疗用品卫生标准以及消毒与灭菌标准。

3）穴位埋线部位消毒：根据不同皮肤消毒剂的使用要求在施术部位由中心向外环形消毒，直径大于 5 厘米。

5. 操作步骤

1）消毒。术者及助手首先戴口罩、帽子，双手按外科手术洗手规范洗手。

2）打开埋线包及外科缝线包，戴无菌手套。

3）将外科缝线剪取 1.0 厘米左右长度的线体备用。

4）一次性使用埋线针。

5）助手对所选择的穴位进行准确定位后，对患者穴位局部消毒。

6）取一段适当长度（1.0 厘米左右）的可吸收性外科缝线，置入一次性注线针的前端，线头勿超出注射针头。

7）用一手拇指和食指固定拟进针穴位，另一只手持针刺入。

8）选择适当针刺方向刺入所需的深度后，边推针芯边退针管，将线体埋植在穴位的肌层或皮下组织内。

9）拔针后用无菌干棉签按压针孔止血，再用医用敷料贴无菌贴敷。

6. 注意事项

1）严格遵守无菌操作，埋线后 6 小时内局部禁止接触水，创面应保持干燥、清洁，防止感染。

2）若发生晕针，应立即停止治疗，按照晕针对症处理。

3）穴位埋线时，如有线体露出皮肤外，一定要拔出，重新定位、消毒和操作。

4）穴位埋线后 3 天内禁止进行剧烈运动，防止埋线部位出现肿胀。

5）穴位埋线后 1 周内尽量减少海鲜等高蛋白质饮食，防止埋线后过敏反应的发生，埋线后若出现硬结反应则慎用再次埋线。

6）每次埋线前都要对患者进行埋线前评估，排除不适宜埋线的患者或暂时不需要埋线的患者。

第三章　中医养生适宜技术操作规范

　　中医养生是在中医理论的指导下，有意识地根据人体生长衰老不可逆的量、质变化规律，所进行的一切物质和精神的身心养护活动。

　　做养生适宜技术操作者的准备和知识储备如下：

一、首诊信息采集（操作前）

　　问诊：了解并记录患者基本情况，包括姓名、年龄、身高、体重、联系方式、家庭住址，详细询问患者病情并记录患者的主诉、现病史、既往史、家族史、过敏史等，有特殊情况者给予记录并用红笔标注。详细记录患者血压、心率、血糖情况，用红笔标记。有手术史者，要详细记录，并用红笔标记，手术史不到一年者不宜治疗。

　　望诊：记录患者面色，舌象（舌苔、舌质，有无齿痕、裂纹等）。

　　切诊：记录患者脉象；给予必要的触诊，记录背部触诊情况，压痛、触痛等情况。

　　闻诊：闻声音，闻气味。有特殊情况者给予记录。肺部有疾患者必要时给予听诊器听诊，并记录。

　　体格检查：根据患者不同疼痛的部位，做相关的体格检查，并且根据影像资料做出相关的初步诊断。

　　通过信息采集，"四诊合参"对患者病情及体质给出诊断。

二、禁忌证

　　明确中医养生适宜技术的适应证和禁忌证，是每一个操作者应该掌握的知识，常见中医养生适宜技术的禁忌证如下：

1）感染性疾病或急、慢性传染病，如丹毒、骨髓炎、急性肝炎、肺结核等。

2）有出血倾向者，如血友病或外伤出血者。

3）操作区域有烫伤、皮肤病或化脓性感染的患者。

4）急性脊柱损伤诊断不明者或者不稳定性脊柱骨折以及脊柱重度滑脱的患者。

5）肌腱或韧带完全或部分断裂。

6）妊娠妇女的腰骶部、臀部和腹部禁用手法；女性在月经期禁用或慎用经筋推拿。

7）精神病患者或骨折、关节脱位，受术者对手法有恐惧心理而不予配合者。

8）不明原因的腹部膨隆、肝内胆管结石、泌尿系统结石、急腹症等不宜实施脊柱推拿，以免贻误病情或者造成损伤。

9）软组织局部肿胀严重者，应查明有无其他合并病症，如骨折、单纯的急性软组织损伤，早期应慎用手法。

10）操作后症状加重或出现异常反应者，应查明原因后再考虑是否继续施术。

11）患有严重内科疾患或年老体弱不能耐受手法施术者；过饥过饱、过度劳累、醉酒之人慎用手法。

三、知识储备

从事中医养生适宜技术者需要有基础的中医知识储备，其中与各个项目相关的知识为一级知识储备，将放在每个项目中予以介绍，二级、三级知识储备为项目共同的知识储备，详述如下：

（一）二级知识储备

1. 中医基础知识

（1）《中医基础理论》：中医学的哲学基础，包括精、气、血、津液，脏象学说，经络学说，体质，病因，病机，防治原则等。

（2）《中医诊断学》：中医诊断的基本原理、中医诊断的基本原则、望诊，闻诊，问诊，切诊，八纲辨证，病性辨证，脏腑辨证，六经辨证等。

（3）《经络腧穴学》：经络概述，腧穴概述，十二经络与腧穴，奇经八脉与腧穴，奇穴，经络的纵横关系，经络的现代研究。

（4）《推拿学》：推拿简史、推拿的作用原理，推拿的治疗原则及方法，推拿常用的诊断方法，推拿手法。

2.西医理论知识（以解剖学为主）

（1）骨学：脊柱的组成、生理弯曲，各部椎骨的特点（颈椎、胸椎、腰椎），椎骨间的连结（椎体间的连结、椎弓间的连结）。

（2）肌学：背部主要肌肉的位置、起止点、作用（斜方肌、背阔肌、竖脊肌等）。

（3）神经系：神经系的基本功能，脊髓节段与椎骨的位置关系，脊神经各神经丛的位置、支配区域。

（4）疾病：颈椎病的概念、分型、治疗方法，腰椎间盘突出症的概念、分型、治疗方法。

（二）三级知识储备（四诊合参，辨证治疗）

《中医内科学》《伤寒论》《金匮要略》《内经》《推拿治疗学》《针灸治疗学》《西医诊断学基础》《内科学》等。

第一节　经筋推拿

一、项目名称

经筋推拿项目是运用中医推拿手法，通过循经点按穴位及特定部位，以达到调理亚健康目的的传统疗法。

二、项目功能

修复损伤组织，疏通阻滞经络，调整脊柱关节紊乱，调和脏腑功能。

三、适应证

适用于颈肩部僵硬酸痛、背腰部及下肢疼痛、疲劳综合征等。

四、标准技术操作规程

1.准备工作

（1）施术者操作前准备：施术者做好个人卫生（包括剪指甲），消毒双手，衣帽整齐，戴口罩。

（2）物品准备：治疗车1辆。①上层。治疗盘1个，盘中放刮痧板1个（刮痧者）；酒精灯、打火机、止血钳各1个，95%酒精棉球、适量罐具；蜡泥1份（蜡泥灸者）；适量艾条（艾灸者）。②下层。床单1条，毛巾（30厘米×70厘米）2条，浴巾1条，养生服1套。

（3）患者准备：换上养生服，取俯卧位于治疗床上。

2. 开始操作　无特殊说明，每个手法操作3遍。

第1步，推督脉、膀胱经、胆经，分推背部。以督脉为中线，双手从颈椎向腰椎做单方向的推法，同法操作于膀胱经和胆经。（5分钟）

第2步，按揉膀胱经、竖脊肌、斜方肌，拿揉小腿。手法以双掌重叠掌根揉法和前臂揉法为主。（5分钟）

第3步，从冈上肌到肩胛骨内侧用小鱼际滚法操作，肩胛骨以下用前臂滚法操作。及时询问患者受力程度，调整手法的力度。（5分钟）

第4步，拇指点按夹脊穴，点背部穴位（包括肩井穴、肺俞穴、心俞穴等五脏背俞穴）。双拇指交替点按，点按穴位频率与患者呼吸节律相同，每个穴位点按3秒。（7分钟）

第5步，弹拨颈肩部、背部阳性反应点。全身放松，疏通经络；病灶点用理筋手法。重点是根据患者的主诉，查找阳性反应点，弹拨附近的肌肉及软组织。（8分钟）

第6步，根据患者情况选取合适的疗法，如拔罐、刮痧、蜡泥灸等。（15分钟）

五、工作语言规范

1. 治疗前　先生（女士）您好！欢迎您来到××，我是您的调理医师××，很高兴为您服务。咱们今天做的是经筋推拿项目。经筋推拿项目可以修复损伤组织，疏通阻滞经络，调整脊柱关节紊乱。另外通过辨证调理背俞穴，达到调和和坚固脏腑的目的。

治疗时间是60分钟，您需要去一下洗手间吗？（不去）

先生（女士），房间温度和光线可以吗？您需要换上养生服，我帮您把衣服挂在衣架上，请您在这张床上取俯卧位。

2. 治疗中　以下按步骤操作并配合语言艺术。

您平时哪里有不舒服吗？我可以根据您的情况给予辨证调理。

第1步，推督脉，膀胱经，胆经，分推背部。首先给您缓解一下肌肉的紧张，您感觉这个力度怎么样？在我手法操作过程中您感觉哪里不舒服请您及时与我沟通。

第2步，按揉膀胱经、竖脊肌、斜方肌，拿揉小腿。这步手法按揉膀胱经和竖脊肌。膀胱经是人体最长的经络，人体每个脏腑在膀胱经第一侧线上都有一个背俞穴，背俞穴是脏腑之气输注于背腰部的穴位。背俞穴与脏腑有特殊关系，在临床上能反映脏腑的虚实盛衰。我们通过辨证选取背俞穴调理，可以达到调理整体的作用。若脊柱椎体有错位，触诊时棘突会有明显压痛、叩击痛或偏歪，棘突周围软组织可有不同程度的紧张甚至痉挛，触之常可感觉有条索样物，压之疼痛。通过理筋手法可达到疏通经络、改善局部循环、促进受损组织修复的作用。

第3步，是肩颈部调理。现代人伏案工作较多，肩颈部是最容易疲劳的部位，初期会有颈肩部疼痛，休息后缓解，但是如果长期疲劳工作，就会形成颈椎病。通过我们的专业手法，可以有效地预防和治疗因颈椎病引起的头痛、头晕、耳鸣、眼花等不适症状。

3. **调理中**

（1）蜡泥灸：先生（女士），经筋推拿项目已经做完，根据您的情况，您的体质偏于阳虚质，适合做的疗法是蜡泥灸，蜡泥灸巧妙地将中药止痛散与加热后的石蜡混合于一体，具有活血、止痛、祛风除湿的多重功效，能迅速温通人体经络，祛风寒除湿邪等，达到快速调理顽疾的目的。它和经筋推拿项目结合，可以起到事半功倍的效果。

（2）拔罐：先生（女士），经筋推拿项目已经做完，根据您的情况，背部结节较多，经络不通，给您运用拔罐疗法，走罐疏通背部膀胱经，并在病变反应处留罐10～15分钟（出痧：根据出痧情况给予进一步解释）。

（3）刮痧：先生（女士），经筋推拿项目已经做完，根据您的情况，背部结节较多，内热比较重，给您运用刮痧疗法，清热祛瘀，疏通经络（出痧：根据出痧情况给予进一步解释）。

（4）艾灸：先生（女士），经筋推拿项目已经做完，根据您的情况，选用艾灸疗法，艾灸具有补阳益气活血、祛寒除湿的多重功效，能迅速温通人体经络，祛风寒除湿邪等。

4. **结束语**　先生（女士），经筋推拿项目到此就做完了，谢谢您积极的配合。如果您有什么意见和建议请告诉我们，我们一定积极改进。

六、注意事项

1）施术前注意房间光线和温度是否合适。

2）诊疗时间约60分钟，手法施术时间以30分钟为宜，不宜太长；有心脏病史、颈椎、腰椎手术史不足2年者，手法以轻柔为主，并询问患者感受，调整手法。

3）注意用毛巾包好患者头发，以免通络油滴到头发上，拔罐时注意保护头发，以免发生事故。

4）嘱患者6小时内不洗澡。

七、终末处理

1. *患者*　治疗结束应嘱患者避免受凉，多饮温开水，当天不做剧烈运动。等患者整理好衣物后将其引领至大厅，嘱其休息5～10分钟，喝温开水或养生药茶1杯。

2. *治疗车及物品整理*

1）治疗车清理干净，放于治疗室指定位置。

2）拔罐治疗结束后，应把酒精灯、止血钳、棉球等归位，火罐用清水清洗后放入消毒液中浸泡消毒1小时，取出晾干备用。

3）刮痧治疗结束后，先用流动水清洗刮痧板，必要时使用清洁剂去除油渍等附着物，做到清洁无污染。依据刮痧器具的不同材质，选择适宜的方式进行清洗消毒处理，达到高水平消毒。消毒方法和消毒剂选用要符合国家标准。可采用含有效氯500～1 000毫克/升的溶液，浸泡至少30分钟。砭石等圆钝用于按压操作的器具，达到中等消毒水平即可，可使用75%酒精、碘类消毒剂、氯己定、季胺盐类等擦拭消毒。遇到器具被污染时应及时去除污染物，再清洁消毒。刮痧器具如被血液、体液污染时，应及时去除污染物，再用含有效氯2 000～5 000毫克/升消毒液，浸泡至少30分钟，清水冲洗，干燥保存。有条件的机构可交由消毒供应中心清洗消毒灭菌。刮痧板用酒精擦洗消毒，晾干后备用，并放入清洁容器内干燥保存，容器每周清洁消毒1次，遇有污染时要随时清洁消毒。

4）整理房间及床单元(床单元一般指医院内一张病床所包含的基本物品：床单、浴巾、毛巾等）。

八、应急预案

1. *通络油过敏*　拔罐或刮痧时用通络油过敏者，应立即停用所用通络油，过敏症状轻者以温水擦洗患处，改用荷荷巴油（霍霍巴油）继续治疗；重者立即停止治疗，用温水擦洗患处，并给予抗过敏治疗。

2. 拔罐起疱　水疱直径小于 5 毫米者，不予特殊处理，日常活动中注意不要把水疱蹭破。水疱大于 5 毫米者，局部消毒，用针灸针或注射器针头刺破水疱下端，用棉签挤出疱液，聚维酮碘消毒患处，嘱患者日常生活中注意保护创面。并注意忌食辛辣刺激食物及发物。

3. 艾灸起疱　参照　拔罐起疱　处理方法。

4. 经筋推拿项目后肌肉疼痛　告知患者可进行热敷处理，并适当休息，近期减少疼痛部位刺激。

九、知识储备（与流程有关的知识点）

一级知识储备

1）中医整体观念的理解，背部调理的重要性。

2）背部经脉的循行路线、背俞穴穴位的定位、主治功能。

3）阳性反应点的寻找以及相对应的临床表现。

4）颈肩部疾病的症状和治疗的重要性。

5）胸椎、腰椎疾病的症状和治疗的重要性。

6）肩井穴、天宗穴等穴位的定位、主治功能及其在整体调理中的重要性。

7）脊柱的解剖结构，生理功能和生理特点。

8）阴阳学说的基本内容及其在中医学中的应用。

十、经筋推拿操作评分标准

经筋推拿操作评分标准见下表。

经筋推拿操作评分标准

项目总分 100 分	要　　求	分值	评分说明	扣分
素质要求 5 分	仪表大方，举止端庄，态度和蔼，衣帽整齐，洗手，戴口罩	5	根据完成情况酌情扣分	

项目总分100分		要 求	分值	评分说明	扣分
操作前准备25分	告知	治疗所需时间、作用，操作方法，局部可能出现的症状等，取得患者合作	4	根据告知情况酌情扣分	
	评估	（四诊）现病史，既往史，家族史，过敏史，是否妊娠或月经期；施术部位皮肤情况、对疼痛的耐受度等	10	根据评估情况酌情扣分	
	物品	治疗车1辆。上层：治疗盘1个，盘中放刮痧板1个（刮痧者）；酒精灯、打火机、止血钳各1个，95%酒精棉球、合适的罐具（拔罐者）各适量；蜡泥1份（蜡泥灸者）；艾条（艾灸者）适量 下层：床单1条，毛巾（30厘米×70厘米）2条，浴巾1条，养生服1套	5	物品准备不完善酌情扣分	
	患者及环境	询问患者治疗前准备情况，取合理体位，松解衣物 室内整洁，保护隐私，注意保暖，避免对流风	6	两项各占3分，回答不完善可酌情扣分	
操作过程40分	核对医嘱	核对姓名、诊断等	3	未核对扣3分；内容不全面酌情扣分	
	操作	按标准技术操作规程步骤操作（步骤附后，详写分值）	25	按表后详细分值评分	
	观察	治疗过程中询问患者感受：舒适度、疼痛情况；观察施术部位皮肤情况	7	未与患者沟通扣7分；内容不全面酌情扣分	
	治疗后	询问患者感受并告知相关注意事项；协助患者取舒适体位	5	未告知注意事项扣3分，未安置体位扣2分	
操作后20分	整理	整理床单元，整理用物，物品清洗消毒并归位，洗手	5	整理不完善酌情扣分	
	评价	操作部位准确，手法操作娴熟，与患者沟通良好，患者感觉达到预期目的	5	评价内容不完善酌情扣分	
	病历记录	详细病历记录治疗情况，签名	2	未记录扣2分；记录不完全扣1分	
	操作后处置	用物按《医疗机构消毒技术规范》处理	8	处置方法不正确，每项扣2分	
理论提问10分		经筋推拿的相关知识 经筋推拿的操作注意事项	10	回答不全面每题扣2分；未答出每题扣5分	

总分：

主考老师签名：　　　　　　　考核日期：　　　年　　月　　日

附　操作步骤及评分分值：

第1步，推督脉、膀胱经、胆经，分推背部。（3分）

第2步，按揉膀胱经、竖脊肌、斜方肌，拿小腿。（3分）

第3步，从冈上肌到肩胛骨内侧用小鱼际滚法操作，肩胛骨以下用前臂滚法操作。（3分）

第4步，拇指点按夹脊穴，点背部穴位。（5分）

第5步，弹拨颈肩部，背部反应点，重点阳性反应点弹拨。（6分）

第6步，根据患者情况选取合适的疗法，如拔罐、刮痧、蜡泥灸等。（5分）

第二节　脊柱调理

一、项目名称

脊柱调理项目是通过手法疏通督脉、膀胱经，并点按背俞穴来调理脏腑功能失调的疗法。

二、项目功能

疏通督脉，提升阳气；疏通膀胱经，调整脊柱关节问题，改善脊柱及其周围肌肉功能，重建脊柱关节平衡；通过辨证调理背俞穴、调理脏腑功能失调。

三、适应证

适用于肩背疼痛、免疫功能紊乱、生理功能低下、慢性疲劳综合征等。

四、标准技术操作规程

1. 准备工作

（1）施术者操作前准备：施术者做好个人卫生（包括剪指甲），消毒双手，衣帽整齐，戴口罩。

（2）物品准备：治疗车1辆。①上层：取一直径30厘米左右，深15～20厘米的器皿，加入10滴减压精油、温度60℃左右温水1 500毫升；通络油1瓶(10～30毫升)。治疗盘1个，放刮痧板1个（刮痧者）；酒精灯、打火机、止血钳各1个，95%酒精棉球、合适的罐具各适量（拔罐者）；蜡泥1份（蜡泥灸者）；艾条适量（艾灸者）。②下层：床单1条，毛巾（30厘米×70厘米）3条，浴巾1条，养生服1套。

（3）患者准备：嘱患者换上养生服，取俯卧位于治疗床上，露出整个背部及腰骶部到八髎穴位置，上肢放于身体两侧，医者取一毛巾压于患者裤腰边缘（毛巾1/4宽压于衣服内，以免治疗油弄脏衣服），再取一毛巾置于裤腰处（热敷时用此毛巾盖背）。

2. 开始操作　无特殊说明，每个手法操作3遍。

第1步，热敷。医者站于床一侧，与患者沟通后，把毛巾放入温水，充分浸湿后，挤出多余水分，以拧不出水为度，用手背试水温后，毛巾充分展开热敷患者整个背部，并配合双掌沿毛巾对角线方向拉伸整个背部。拉两遍后，先将毛巾上下1/4折叠再对折，一手取下热敷毛巾，另一手顺势用备好的毛巾盖于背部，以保存温度。（1分钟）

第2步，铺油，整个背部安抚（安抚即放松的按摩手法）。①医者站于床头，取适量通络油在掌心处，双掌相对搓（以双手掌蘸满通络油但不滴下为度，不能滴到患者背部、头发及床单上），双掌分开放于脊柱两侧膀胱经，由大椎穴水平开始，按照掌根→掌心→指部→指尖的次序充分贴于背部，然后按以上顺序抬离背部（除拇指外其余四指指尖不离开背部），再按照以上顺序重复贴于背部、抬离背部，直至腰骶部，使双掌经过之背部铺满通络油。②抬起双手，双掌指尖相对紧贴于背部放于脊柱两侧，由大椎穴水平向下平推至腰骶部，然后转掌与脊柱平行，回拉至大椎穴水平，双掌相离至肩部包肩，顺着斜方肌的走行提拉至风池穴，中指点按风池穴。

特别提示：背部安抚若患者背部面积较大，可重复以上动作1次，以背部铺满通络油但无多余通络油流动为度。（1分钟）

第3步，疏通督脉推八髎。双手拇指相邻于脊柱垂直方向放于督脉上，其余四指指尖向外贴于背部，拇指从大椎穴开始用力推督脉至腰骶部八髎区，（可直推也可分段推）推过后可背部安抚1～2遍。（2分钟）

第4步，在督脉上走"8"字。双手拇指相邻与脊柱垂直方向放于督脉上，拇指交替由棘突上沿棘突侧面划弧线至棘突下，双拇指交替推至第五腰椎棘突下。（2分钟）

第5步，拇指推夹脊穴。双手拇指直推双侧夹脊穴，也可分段推，有结节或条索的地方可重点疏通（拇指推或点按）。推至腰骶部，拇指交替弧形推八髎区。（2

分钟）

第6步，拇指推膀胱经。操作同第5步，施术于膀胱经第一侧线。（2分钟）

第7步，双拳半握疏通膀胱经。双手半握拳以指间关节为着力点，分别疏通脊柱两侧膀胱经，有结节或条索的地方可重复推。（2分钟）

第8步，提捏颈部点穴位（大椎穴、风池穴、风府穴）。医者蹲于床头处，双手拿揉肩部，之后转为站立位，转手，双手拇指重叠，点按大椎穴，双手包肩用双手虎口处提拉肩井穴区域，然后提拉斜方肌至后枕部，中指分别点按两侧风池穴，再重叠点按风府穴。（2分钟）

第9步，双手拨肩排毒素。双手拇指推肩部肌肉，由肩髎穴向内推至大椎穴后转手掌根瞬间发力斜向外下推下。（1分钟）

第10步，回手揉按双颈肩。回手，双手半握拳，指间关节着力，提拉肩部由肩髎穴到大椎穴，然后施术于颈部两侧肌肉。（2分钟）

第11步，太极揉按转大椎。双手拇指太极式转按大椎穴区域。（1分钟）

第12步，两秒间点夹脊穴。双拇指点按夹脊穴，每穴点按2秒；点穴后背部安抚。（2分钟）

第13步，回手拉抹揉肩胛。上一步最后一遍背部安抚后，掌根由肩部转手下至双侧肩胛下角，双掌根相对用力，挤按肩胛区肌肉，提拉至大椎穴处。（1分钟）

第14步，反手轮转调肝脾。上一步做完后顺势向下，提拉肝俞、胆俞区域至大椎穴处，再向下，提拉脾俞、胃俞区域至大椎穴。（1分钟）

第15步，马鞍双点肾俞穴。右手拇指、食指马鞍式点按肾俞穴。（1分钟）

第16步，太极轮转养命门。以命门穴为中心，双掌太极式施术于肾区。（1分钟）

第17步，双手重叠通三焦。双手重叠，右手在下，双手同时用力，以右掌根为主，由大椎穴推督脉直至腰骶部，双手分开分别由两侧膀胱经上拉至肩部。（2分钟）

第18步，左右拉抹调阴阳。双掌放于脊柱两侧膀胱经，一侧由肩向下推至腰骶部，另一侧由腰骶部向上拉至肩部，两侧同时操作，调整阴阳，操作8～10遍。（2分钟）

第19步，回手搓抹热经络。双手重叠由下向上搓热督脉（频率120～160次/分），先搓热肾区再向上延伸，直至搓热整个督脉。（1分钟）

第20步，全身放松大排毒。背部按抚，沿肩部斜方肌向手臂方向推，经上臂

外侧到肘关节再推至前臂内侧，向下推至指尖排毒。（1分钟）

手法操作后根据患者情况选择适合的疗法，如拔罐、刮痧、蜡泥灸等。（15分钟）

五、工作语言规范

1. 治疗前　先生（女士）您好！欢迎您来到××，我是您的调理医师××，很高兴为您服务！咱们今天做的是脊柱调理项目，脊柱调理项目可以疏通督脉，提升阳气；疏通膀胱经，调理脊柱功能异常造成的疼痛和内脏疾病。

治疗时间大概需要60分钟，您需要去一下洗手间吗？（不去）

先生（女士），房间温度和光线可以吗？您需要把上衣脱掉，我帮您把衣服挂在衣架上，请您在这张床上取俯卧位。

2. 治疗中　以下按步骤操作并配合语言艺术。

你平时哪里有不舒服吗？我可以根据您的情况给予辨证调理。

第1步，热敷。现在先给您背部做个中药液热敷。您感觉药温可以吗？（很好）热敷可以缓解肌肉紧张，药液和温热协同作用，疏通背部经络，为手法治疗起到很好的铺垫作用。

第2步，铺油。通络油是由多种中药提取而成的，有通经络、除寒凉等作用。

第3步，疏通督脉推八髎。现在为您做的是疏通督脉。督脉为阳脉之海，能够激发和提升阳气，可改善阳虚引起的怕冷、手脚冰凉等症状。您感觉力度可以吗？

第4步，在督脉上走"8"字。这一步我可以通过您脊柱棘突的位置，了解您的脊柱情况，以便后面给您选择性调理。

第5步，拇指推夹脊穴。这一步是疏通夹脊。夹脊穴与脏腑密切相关，是体内脏腑与背部体表相联通的点。解剖学上每穴都有相应的脊神经后支及其伴行的动脉、静脉分布，研究认为夹脊穴能调节自主神经的功能，故用夹脊穴治疗与自主神经功能有关的疾病，如血管性头痛、肢端感觉异常症、自主神经功能失调、脑血管病、高血压等。

第6步，拇指推膀胱经。

第7步，双拳半握疏通膀胱经。第6步、第7步手法疏通膀胱经。膀胱经是人体最长的经络，人体每个脏腑在膀胱经第一侧线上都有一个背俞穴，背俞穴是脏腑之气输注与背腰部的穴位。背俞穴与脏腑有特殊关系，在临床上能反映脏腑的虚实盛衰，当背俞穴出现各种异常反应，如结节、条索状物、压痛、丘疹等往往能够反映相关脏腑的异常。我们通过辨证选取背俞穴调理，可以达到调理整体的作用。膀胱经是人体的防御屏障，风、寒、暑、湿等外邪侵袭人体，如果防御功能差，就会引发疾病。调理好膀胱经，能够提升正气，提高人体免疫力。

第8步，提捏颈部点穴位（大椎、风池、风府）。

第9步，双手拨肩排毒素。

第10步，回手揉按双颈肩。

第11步，太极揉按转大椎。

刚做的手法主要是颈肩部调理。现代人伏案工作较多，颈肩部是最容易疲劳的地方，初期会有颈肩部疼痛，休息后缓解，但是如果长期不重视，就会形成颈椎病。通过我们的专业手法，可以有效地预防和治疗因颈椎病引起的头痛、头晕、耳鸣、眼花等不适症状。

第12步，两秒间点夹脊穴。

第13步，回手拉抹揉双肩胛。

第14步，反手轮转调肝脾。

第15步，马鞍双点肾俞穴。肾俞穴是肾脏精气输注于腰部的穴位，肾为先天之本，通过点按肾俞穴，从而达到强腰补肾的作用。

第16步，太极轮转养命门。养命门就是养肾，中医讲肾为先天之本，注重养肾，能够调理腰膝酸软、失眠健忘、神疲乏力。

第17步，双手重叠通三焦。

第18步，左右拉抹调阴阳。现在给您做的是调理阴阳。中医讲阴阳达到动态平衡了才健康，阴平阳秘就是这个意思。

第19步，回手搓抹热经络。

第20步，全身放松大排毒。

3. **调理中** 同本章"第一节经筋推拿"。

4. **结束语** 先生（女士），脊柱调理项目到此就做完了，谢谢您积极的配合。如果您有什么意见和建议请告诉我们，我们一定积极改进。

六、注意事项

1）施术前注意房间光线和温度是否合适。

2）治疗时间约60分钟，手法施术时间以30分钟为宜，不宜太长；有心脏病史，颈椎、腰椎手术史小于2年者，手法以轻柔为主，并询问患者感受，调整手法。

3）注意用毛巾包好患者头发，以免药油滴到头发上，拔罐时注意保护头发，以免发生事故。

4）嘱患者6小时内不洗澡。

七、终末处理

1. 患者　治疗结束应把患者背部通络油擦干净。嘱患者避免受凉，多饮温开水，当天不做剧烈运动。等患者整理好衣物后将其引领至大厅，嘱其休息5～10分钟，喝温开水或养生药茶1杯。

2. 治疗车及物品整理

1）治疗车清理干净，放于治疗室指定位置。

2）拔罐治疗结束后，应把酒精灯、止血钳、棉球等归位，火罐用清水清洗后放入消毒液中浸泡消毒1小时，取出晾干备用。

3）刮痧治疗结束后，刮痧板清洗后，用酒精擦洗消毒，晾干后备用。

4）通知巡视护士整理房间。

八、应急预案

1. 通络油过敏　参照本章第一节"经筋推拿"处理方法。

2. 拔罐起疱　参照本章第一节"经筋推拿"处理方法。

3. 脊柱调理项目治疗后肌肉疼痛　参照本章第一节"经筋推拿"处理方法。

九、知识储备（与流程相关的知识点）

一级知识储备

1）对中医整体观念的理解，背部调理的重要性。

2）背部经脉的循行路线、重点穴位的定位、主治功能。

3）风池穴、风府穴的定位、归经、主治功能。

4）颈肩部疾病的症状和治疗的重要性。

5）胸椎疾病的症状和治疗的重要性。

6）肝与脾的关系。

7）肾俞穴、命门穴命名的由来、穴位定位、主治功能及其在整体调理中的重要性。

8）三焦的含义、生理功能和生理特点。

9）阴阳学说的基本内容及其在中医学中的应用。

十、脊柱调理操作评分标准

脊柱调理操作评分标准见下表。

脊柱调理操作评分标准

项目总分 100 分		要　　求	分值	评分说明	扣分
素质要求 5 分		仪表大方，举止端庄，态度和蔼，衣帽整齐，洗手，戴口罩	5	根据完成情况酌情扣分	
操作前准备 25 分	告知	治疗所需时间、作用，操作方法，局部可能出现的症状等，取得患者合作	4	根据告知情况酌情扣分	
	评估	（四诊）现病史，既往史，家族史，过敏史，是否妊娠或月经期；施术部位皮肤情况、对疼痛的耐受度等	10	根据评估情况酌情扣分	
	物品	治疗车 1 辆。上层：器皿 1 个，精油 1 瓶，通络油 1 瓶，治疗盘 1 个，盘中放刮痧板 1 个（刮痧者）；酒精灯、打火机、止血钳各 1 个，95% 酒精棉球、合适的罐具（拔罐者）各适量；蜡泥（蜡泥灸者）1 份；艾条（艾灸者）适量 下层：床单 1 条，毛巾（30 厘米 ×70 厘米）3 条，浴巾 1 条，养生服 1 套	5	物品准备不完善酌情扣分	
	患者及环境	询问患者治疗前准备情况，取合理体位，松解衣物 室内整洁，保护隐私，注意保暖，避免对流风	6	两项各占 3 分，回答不完善可酌情扣分	
操作过程 40 分	核对医嘱	核对姓名、诊断等	3	未核对扣 3 分；内容不全面酌情扣分	
	操作	按标准技术操作规程步骤操作（步骤附后，详写分值）	25	按表后详细分值评分	
	观察	治疗过程中询问患者感受：舒适度、疼痛情况；观察施术部位皮肤情况	7	未与患者沟通扣 7 分；内容不全面酌情扣分	
	治疗后	询问患者感受并告知相关注意事项；协助患者取舒适体位	5	未告知注意事项扣 3 分，未安置体位扣 2 分	

项目总分 100分		要　求	分值	评分说明	扣分
操作后 20分	整理	整理床单元，整理用物，物品清洗消毒并归位，洗手	5	整理不完善酌情扣分	
	评价	操作部位准确，手法操作娴熟，与患者沟通良好，患者感觉达到预期目的	5	评价内容不完善酌情扣分	
	病历记录	详细病历记录治疗情况，签名	2	未记录扣2分；记录不完全扣1分	
	操作后处置	用物按《医疗机构消毒技术规范》处理	8	处置方法不正确，每项扣2分	
理论提问 10分		脊柱调理的相关知识脊柱调理的操作注意事项	10	回答不全面每项扣2分；未答出每题扣5分	

总分：

主考老师签名：　　　　　　　　　考核日期：　　　　　年　　月　　日

附　操作步骤及评分分值：

第1步，热敷。（1分）

第2步，铺油，整个背部安抚。（1分）

第3步，疏通督脉推八髎。（1分）

第4步，在督脉上走"8"字。（1分）

第5步，拇指推夹脊穴。（1分）

第6步，拇指推膀胱经。（1分）

第7步，双拳半握疏通膀胱经。（1分）

第8步，提捏颈部点穴位（大椎穴、风池穴、风府穴）。（1分）

第9步，双手拨肩排毒素。（1分）

第10步，回手揉按双颈肩。（1分）

第11步，太极揉按转大椎。（1分）

第12步，两秒间点夹脊穴。（1分）

第13步，回手拉抹揉肩胛。（1分）

第14步，反手轮转调肝脾。（1分）

第15步，马鞍双点肾俞穴。（1分）

第16步，太极轮转养命门。（1分）

第17步，双手重叠通三焦。（1分）

第18步，左右拉抹调阴阳。（1分）

第19步，回手搓抹热经络。（1分）

第20步，全身放松大排毒。（1分）

手法操作后根据患者情况选择适合的疗法，如拔罐、刮痧、蜡泥灸等。（5分）

第三节　国药养颜

一、项目名称

国药养颜项目是运用国术点穴配合精油刮痧和纯中药面膜，改善面部肤色暗沉、皮肤干燥、皱纹等问题的疗法。

二、项目功能

疏通面部经络，改善面部血液循环，提亮肤色，减少细纹，延缓衰老。

三、适应证

适用于面色萎黄、色斑、皮肤干燥、松弛、皱纹增多等。

四、禁忌证

1）面部对中药过敏者慎用。

2）面部有外伤或有皮炎、疱疹等皮肤问题者禁用。

3）面部做过双眼皮、隆鼻、垫下巴等微整形手术不足半年者。

五、标准技术操作规程

1. 准备工作

（1）施术者操作前准备：施术者做好个人卫生（包括剪指甲），消毒双手，衣帽整齐，戴口罩。

（2）物品准备：治疗车1辆。①上层。治疗盘1个，盘中放面部卸妆乳、眼唇部卸妆液、洁面乳、按摩膏、精油各1瓶，面膜1张，柔肤水或爽肤水、精华液、日霜或晚霜、隔离霜各1瓶，面部刮痧板1个，棉签、化妆棉各适量，面巾1张。②中层。器皿（直径30厘米，深15～20厘米）1个，床单1条，毛巾（30厘米

×70厘米）3条，浴巾1条，养生服1套。③下层。温水壶、污水桶各1个。

（3）患者准备：换好养生服，取仰卧位躺在美容床上，充分暴露面部，盖上浴巾，然后用毛巾包头。

2. 开始操作　无特殊说明，每个手法操作3遍。

（1）洁面（7分钟）：

第1步，卸妆。用棉签蘸眼唇部卸妆液卸眼唇部妆，用化妆棉和面部卸妆液卸面部妆。

第2步，用面巾在患者额头试水温，然后擦拭整个面部。操作步骤：右侧内眼角依次由眼睛、眉毛、额头、鼻子、脸颊三线、下巴到耳朵；换面巾另一面，擦左侧半边脸（顺序同右侧）。

第3步，洁面乳五点式（即额头、两颊、鼻子、下巴）打开。

第4步，洁面无特殊说明，均用中指和无名指操作。操作步骤：①额头。由额头中间分别向外侧打圈至太阳穴结束。②眼部。依次由目外眦、下眼睑、目内眦、眉毛、太阳穴顺序操作。③鼻部。鼻头从内向外打圈，然后点按迎香穴，然后提拉地仓穴经迎香穴到睛明穴。④唇周。双手中指交替"C"形洗唇部周围皮肤。⑤脸颊。脸颊分三线从内向外打圈操作。三线：从承浆穴打圈至听会穴；从地仓穴打圈到耳前听宫穴；从迎香穴打圈至太阳穴。⑥脖子。双手四指交替向上提拉3～5遍，然后洗耳朵。⑦结束。用面巾清洁面部，拍爽肤水或柔肤水。

（2）按摩（16分钟）：按摩膏五点式打开，然后按步骤操作。

第1步，额部。①双手中指和无名指分别从中间向两边打圈至太阳穴。②双手虎口由印堂穴向前发际方向拉抹额部中间区域。③双掌根交替拉抹整个额部。④双手中指和无名指交替提拉"川"字纹。⑤双手交替"C"形拉开额横纹。⑥双掌根按压额头中间部分区域，结束。

第2步，眼部。①双手中指和无名指在眼部周围由外向内环形按摩眼周围皮肤。②左手四指指腹由右目内眦向外上方提拉眼部皮肤至太阳穴，右手掌根顺势亦提拉至太阳穴。然后同法操作于左侧。③左手食指和中指呈手剪刀状，从右目内眦向外上方提拉眼部皮肤至太阳穴，右手掌根顺势亦提拉至太阳穴。然后同法操作于左侧。④左手食指和中指分别置于右侧上、下眼睑处，右手中指和无名指从外向内打圈按揉眼袋至目内眦。⑤搓热双手热敷双侧眼部。

第3步，鼻部。手法同"洁面"第4步操作。

第 4 步，唇部。点唇部周围穴位（人中穴、承浆穴、地仓穴）然后双手中指交替 "C" 形按摩唇部周围皮肤。

第 5 步，脸颊。①分别取四指指腹、大鱼际、指间关节为着力点，按洁面时的 "三线" 按摩面部皮肤。②双手四指指腹轮弹双侧脸颊。③双手包脸，先右侧后左侧。④抬下颌。双手中指和无名指垂直向头顶方向抬下颌，然后双拇指协助下颌恢复原位。⑤双手五指交叉分别从额部、眼睛、鼻翼两侧、上唇、下颌五线由中间向两侧斜向上提拉面部→双手拇指和食指搓揉双侧耳，弹耳结束。⑥用面巾清洁面部，拍爽肤水或柔肤水。

（3）刮痧（15 分钟）：

第 1 步，打开精油。精油五点式打开，然后双手持刮痧板把精油均匀地布满面部皮肤。

第 2 步，查找结节。双手持刮痧板与面部皮肤成 45° 角，查找步骤：①右手持刮痧板用刮痧板一角刮两眉之间，额部分别从督脉刮至两侧发际。②双手持刮痧板提拉睛明穴后刮双侧眉棱骨，斜向上刮至发际。③从下眼睑开始刮，经颧上、太阳穴斜向上刮至发际。④从迎香穴经颧骨（轻刮）斜向上刮至耳前听宫穴。⑤从迎香穴经颧下刮至听会穴。⑥刮鼻子。⑦从人中穴经颊车穴刮至耳根。⑧从承浆穴刮至耳根。⑨用刮痧板边缘着力刮下颌至耳后。

第 3 步，按揉结节。双手持刮痧板与皮肤成 30° 角，步骤同第 2 步，在结节处用刮痧板按揉半分钟，无结节处按步骤刮拭。

第 4 步，梳理面部。双手持刮痧板按第 2 步中步骤刮整个面部，结束。用面巾清洁面部，拍爽肤水或柔肤水。

（4）敷面膜（17 分钟）：

第 1 步，调面膜。用蜂蜜和纯净水调中药面膜，调成稀糊状（以涂到面部不干也不流下为度），面膜、蜂蜜、纯净水各 15 克。

第 2 步，敷面膜。将面膜均匀涂于面部，留 15 分钟。

（5）敷面膜期间做头、颈、肩部手法放松：

第 1 步，头部。①右手拇指点按督脉神庭穴至百会穴。②双手拇指点按两侧膀胱经（头部循行部位）。③用双手指腹抓揉头部。④用双手指间隙顺头发。⑤用空拳扣头部督脉、膀胱经、胆经。⑥用双手指腹拿揉头部。

第 2 步，颈部。①右手指腹揉后枕部。②右手指腹揉项韧带及夹脊穴。③右手虎口提拉颈部至风池穴。

第3步，肩部。①双手揉按斜方肌。②双手向下推按肩部。③双掌根按云门穴区。④双手揉拿上臂。⑤双手空拳叩上臂。

（6）去面膜（5分钟）：用面巾洁面后，拍爽肤水或柔肤水，搽乳液、精华液、眼霜、日霜、隔离霜。

六、工作语言规范

1. **治疗前**　先生（女士）您好！欢迎您来到××，我是您的调理医师××，很高兴为您服务。咱们今天做的是国药养颜项目。国药养颜项目可以改善面部血液循环，调理面部色斑、皮肤晦暗等问题。

治疗时间大概需要60分钟，您需要去一下洗手间吗？（不去）

先生（女士），请您换上养生服，在这张床上取仰卧位。我用毛巾给您包一下头，松紧可以吗？我们开始操作吧。

2. **治疗中**　以下按步骤操作并配合语言艺术。

先生（女士），现在给您洁面，先给您卸一下妆，水温可以吗？（可以）

（1）面部按摩：面部按摩可以疏通经络，把面部细小的皱纹提拉开，把面部皮肤做一个提升。①额部。额部的手法可以把额横纹、川字纹拉开，疏通经络，改善局部血液循环。②眼部。眼部手法把眼部皮肤斜向上提拉，把鱼尾纹提拉开，按揉打圈、按揉下眼睑，改善眼部的血液循环，有利于缓解黑眼圈和眼袋。黑眼圈重提示睡眠不好或肾虚，眼袋重提示脾肾阳虚，气血不足，可以通过全身调理来改善眼的局部问题。先生（女士），手法力度可以吗？按摩面颊，可以使面部血液循环改善，皮肤滋润。

（2）面部刮痧：先生（女士），面部刮痧是国药养颜项目的特色部分。在做的过程中可能会有点儿疼，有的地方有结节，把结节按揉开，面部会轻松，如果力度太重的话您跟我说一下。面部是身体的全息区之一，面部有结节的地方也提示了对应脏腑有问题。把面部的结节按揉开对脏腑也有辅助的调理作用（有结节的地方提示的问题给患者予以解释）。先生（女士），您额头这一块儿出了点痧，两天基本上就吸收了，不必太担心。

（3）面膜：先生（女士），这个中药面膜是我们针对面部定制的一款面膜，用蜂蜜和纯净水调和，蜂蜜有保湿滋润皮肤的作用，面膜有益气养血通络功效。先生

（女士），面膜留 15 分钟，留面膜的时间我给您做头部、颈肩部的放松。现在面膜到时间了给您去掉，给您拍爽肤水（柔肤水），搽面霜。

先生（女士），国药养颜项目做完了。您面部气色比之前好多了，皮肤看起来比较通透，您可以看一下（给镜子）。国药养颜是面部的周护理，最好 1 周做 1 次，您看下一次什么时间能做，可以提前跟我们预约。

3. 结束语　先生（女士）国药养颜项目到此就做完了，谢谢您的配合。如果您有什么意见和建议请告诉我们，我们一定积极改进。

七、注意事项

1）施术前注意房间光线和温度是否合适。

2）面部刮痧力度以患者耐受为度，不要太重。

3）施术过程中观察面部是否有过敏症状。

4）如不慎将面膜入眼，应及时冲洗。

5）头颈部注意用毛巾包好，以防止精油沾染头发和衣服上。

八、终末处理

1. 患者　治疗结束为患者做治疗评价，针对患者情况给予简单的养生建议，流程结束嘱其休息 5～10 分钟，喝温开水或养生药茶 1 杯。

2. 治疗车及物品整理

1）治疗车清理干净，放于治疗室指定位置。

2）面部刮痧板清洗后，置于酒精中消毒以备用。

3）整理房间。

九、应急预案

1. 面部精油过敏　立即停用所用精油。过敏症状轻者以温水擦洗患处，重者给予抗过敏治疗。

2. 面膜过敏　立即停用中药面膜。过敏症状轻者以温水擦洗患处，给予患者解释；重者给予抗过敏治疗。

十、知识储备

1. 一级知识储备（与流程有关的知识点）

1）中医整体观念，脾胃与面部的关系。

2）面部的经络循行、面部穴位的定位、主治功能（太阳、睛明、迎香、听宫、地仓等穴的定位）。

3）面部全息区知识，面部结节提示的问题。

4）中药面膜的成分和作用。

5）头部的经络循行及作用。

6）颈肩部疾患的症状及简单治疗。

2. 二级知识储备（基础知识）　《医学美容学》中的第一章绪论、第二章 保健美容、第三章 皮肤美容（重点）。

十一、国药养颜操作评分标准

国药养颜操作评分标准见下表。

国药养颜操作评分标准

项目总分 100分		要　　求	分值	评分说明	扣分
素质要求 5分		仪表大方，举止端庄，态度和蔼，衣帽整齐，洗手，戴口罩	5	根据完成情况酌情扣分	
操作前准备 25分	告知	治疗所需时间、作用，操作方法，局部可能出现的症状等，取得患者合作	4	根据告知情况酌情扣分	
	评估	（四诊）现病史，既往史，家族史，过敏史，是否妊娠或月经期；施术部位皮肤情况、对疼痛的耐受度等	10	根据评估情况酌情扣分	
	物品	治疗车1辆；上层：治疗盘1个，盘中放面部卸妆乳、眼唇部卸妆液、洁面乳、按摩膏、精油各1瓶，面膜1张，柔肤水或爽肤水、精华液、日霜或晚霜、隔离霜各1瓶，面部刮痧板1个，棉签、化妆棉各适量，面巾1张 下层：直径30厘米、深15～20厘米的器皿1个，床单1条，毛巾（30厘米×70厘米）3条，浴巾1条，养生服1套 底层：温水壶、污水桶各1个	5	准备不完善酌情扣分	

项目总分 100 分		要　求	分值	评分说明	扣分
操作过程 40 分	患者及环境	询问患者治疗前准备情况，取合理体位，松解衣物 室内整洁，保护隐私，注意保暖，避免对流风	6	两项各占 3 分，回答不完善可酌情扣分	
	核对医嘱	核对姓名、诊断等	3	未核对扣 3 分；内容不全面酌情扣分	
	操作	按标准技术操作规程步骤操作（步骤附后，详写分值）	25	按表后详细分值评分	
	观察	治疗过程中询问患者感受：舒适度、疼痛情况；观察施术部位皮肤情况	7	未与患者沟通扣 7 分；内容不全面酌情扣分	
	治疗后	询问患者感受并告知相关注意事项；协助患者取舒适体位	5	未告知注意事项扣 3 分，未安置体位扣 2 分	
操作后 20 分	整理	整理床单元，整理用物，物品清洗消毒并归位，洗手	5	整理不完善酌情扣分	
	评价	操作部位准确，手法操作娴熟，与患者沟通良好，患者感觉预期目的达成	5	评价内容不完善酌情扣分	
	病历记录	详细病历记录治疗情况，签名	2	未记录扣 2 分；记录不完全扣 1 分	
	操作后处置	用物按《医疗机构消毒技术规范》处理	8	处置方法不正确，每项扣 2 分	
理论提问 10 分		国药养颜的相关知识 国药养颜中面部刮痧的作用	10	回答不全面每题扣 2 分；未答出每题扣 5 分	

总分：

主考老师签名：　　　　　　　考核日期：　　　年　　月　　日

附　操作步骤及评分分值：

（1）洁面（7 分）：

第 1 步，卸妆。（1 分）

第 2 步，用面巾在患者额头试水温，然后擦拭整个面部。（1 分）

第 3 步，洁面乳五点式打开。（1 分）

第 4 步，洁面。（4 分）

（2）按摩（5 分）：按摩膏五点式打开，然后按步骤操作。

（3）刮痧（5 分）：共 4 步。

（4）面膜（3分）：调面膜，敷面膜。

（5）头、颈、肩部手法放松（3分）：共3步。

（6）去面膜（2分）：按上面的要求进行操作。

第四节　冲脉、任脉、带脉调理

一、项目名称

冲脉、任脉、带脉调理，运用循经推法、运法，配合艾灸疗法调节冲脉、任脉、带脉，调理女性月经不调、痛经、肥胖、胃肠功能紊乱等问题。

二、项目功能

手法疏通腰骶部和腹部经络，补肾气，调冲任，调理脾胃，使气血生化有源，冲脉、任脉、带脉调和，改善女性生殖功能。

三、适应证

适用于卵巢功能早衰、月经不调、痛经、更年期综合征、胃肠功能紊乱等问题。

四、标准技术操作规程

1. 准备工作

（1）施术者操作前准备：施术者做好个人卫生（包括剪指甲），消毒双手，衣帽整齐，戴口罩。

（2）物品准备：治疗车1辆。①上层。取直径30厘米，深15～20厘米的器皿1个，加入10滴精油和温度60℃左右水1 500毫升；通络油1瓶（10～30毫升），酒精灯、打火机各1个，艾条适量。②下层。床单1条，毛巾（30厘米×70厘米）3条，浴巾1条，养生服1套。

（3）患者准备：嘱患者换上养生服，取俯卧位躺着床上，露出背部肾区、腰骶部到八髎区位置，上肢放于身体两侧。术者取2条毛巾分别压在操作部位的上下两边衣服下面。以免通络油弄脏衣服。

2. 开始操作　无特殊说明，每个手法操作3遍。

（1）腰部：

第1步，热敷。术者站于床一侧，与患者沟通后，把毛巾放入温水中，充分浸湿后，挤出多余水分，以拧不出水为度，用手背试水温后，将毛巾对折两层热敷整个肾区及腰骶部，然后将毛巾再对折，一手取下热敷毛巾，另一手顺势用备好的毛巾盖于背部，以保存温度。（1分钟）

第2步，铺油，腰骶部安抚。把通络油均匀地铺在患者腰骶部。术者站于床一侧，取适量通络油在掌心处，双掌相对搓（以双手掌蘸满通络油但不滴下为度，不能滴到患者背部、头发及床单上），双掌分别由脊柱向两侧打圈的方式进行铺油，使双掌经过腰骶部铺满通络油。（1分钟）

第3步，①打开通络油，点肾俞穴、志室穴，反手推八髎区，点按八髎穴，然后腰骶部安抚。②双手拇指点按以上穴位，然后转身向腰部双手拇指交替推八髎区，并点按八髎穴。每遍结束后可进行腰骶部安抚1次。（3分钟）

第4步，①双掌根推带脉4～5次，分推后回手排毒。②双掌根交替从脊柱向外推一侧带脉，然后换另外一侧。重复动作3～5遍，每遍做完可进行腰部安抚1次。(2分钟）

第5步，双手虎口来回推腰部肾区。双手拇指和其余四指分开，用虎口在肾区做上下来回推拉动作。动作要沉着、柔和、力度均匀。推3～5个来回后腰部安抚。（3分钟）

第6步，双手交替提拉带脉然后分推排毒。双手交替提拉一侧带脉10遍，同样方法做另一侧，双手手掌平放于腰部肾区，指尖朝外，掌根相对，分推至带脉再迅速向上提拉，力量的方向最后是集聚至两掌，发出清脆的击掌声。重复以上动作3～5遍。腰骶部安抚。（2分钟）

第7步，搓热肾区及腰骶部安抚，结束。双手重叠贴于皮肤，指尖与脊柱垂直，做快速来回搓肾区及八髎区至发热（10遍），结束。（2分钟）

（2）腹部：

第1步，热敷。术者站于床一侧，与患者沟通后，嘱患者取仰卧位露出巨阙穴至中极穴，在施术部位上、下分别垫上毛巾，把毛巾放入温水中，充分浸湿后，挤出多余水分，以拧不出水为度，用手背试水温后，将毛巾对折两层热敷整个腹部，然后将毛巾进行对折整齐，一手取下热敷毛巾，另一手顺势用施术部位下面的毛巾盖于腹部，以保持温度。（1分钟）

第2步，铺油，腹部安抚。术者站于床一侧，取适量通络油在掌心处，双掌相对搓（以双手掌蘸满油但不滴下为度，不能滴到患者身上、头发及床单上），双掌以打圈的方式在腹部交替进行铺油，使双掌经过的腹部铺满油；操作过程中双手始终紧贴皮肤。若患者腹部面积较大，可重复以上动作1次。（1分钟）

第3步，①顺时针打开通络油，点中脘穴、天枢穴、气海穴、关元穴、中极穴、子宫穴、归来穴，安抚施术区。②以一手中指或拇指为着力点，依次进行点按以上穴位，每穴3～5遍。每遍结束后可进行安抚施术区1次。（3分钟）

第4步，双手掌交替顺任脉由巨阙穴至中极穴，顺双侧胃经由12肋骨游离缘至归来穴。双手手掌紧贴于施术部位，从上至下两掌交替顺任脉（由巨阙穴至中极穴）。同样动作顺双侧胃经，先左后右（由12肋骨游离缘至归来穴）。（3分钟）

第5步，掌心按揉脐上、脐下、脐左、脐右及脐中。（3分钟）

第6步，双手掌交替提拉带脉，双手分推反手排毒。双手掌交替提拉一侧带脉10遍，同样手法施术于另一侧，然后双手手掌平放于腹部施术部位，指尖朝外，掌根相对，分推至带脉再迅速向上提拉，力量最后集聚至两掌，发出清脆的击掌声。腹部安抚。（2分钟）

第7步，双手拉抹带脉10次。双手分别放于腰部两侧，然后做相对力量的提拉，一上一下交替进行拉抹。腹部安抚。（3分钟）

第8步，双手搓热暖子宫穴、神阙穴，根据患者具体情况进行腰部或腹部施灸30分钟。（30分钟）

五、工作语言规范

1.治疗前　女士您好！欢迎您来到××，我是您的调理医师××，很高兴为您服务。咱们今天做的是冲脉、任脉、带脉调理项目，冲脉、任脉、带脉调理项目可以疏通经络、调气活血、调理冲任、暖宫散寒等。冲脉和任脉是奇经八脉中的两脉，中医讲，"冲为血海，任主胞胎"，冲脉、任脉与妇女经、带、孕、胎、产等生理功能有着极为密切的关系，运用循经推法和运法、点穴等手法，调节冲任，可用于女性生理功能及胃肠功能的调理养护等。

治疗时间大概需要60分钟，您需要去一下洗手间吗？（不去）

女士，请您换上养生服，我帮您把衣服挂在衣架上。您先在这张床上取俯卧位。

2. *治疗中* 以下按步骤操作并配合语言艺术。

（1）腰部：

第1步，热敷。现在先给您背部做热敷。你感觉水温可以吗（很好）？热敷可以缓解肌肉紧张，通络油和温热协同作用，疏通背部经络，为手法治疗起到很好的铺垫作用。

第2步，铺油。通络油是由多种中药提取而成的，有通经络、除寒凉等作用。您平时腰部有不舒服，怕冷吗？我可以根据您的个人情况给予辨证调理。

第3步，打开通络油，点肾俞穴、志室穴，反手推三角区，点按八髎穴后腰骶部安抚。现在为您做的是点穴位。腰为肾之府，肾主生殖，很多腰部酸痛、怕冷、月经紊乱等都跟肾脏功能失调有关，肾俞穴是肾脏精气输注于腰部的穴位，肾为先天之本，点按肾俞穴，有强腰补肾的作用，肾俞穴是调理肾脏功能的重要的穴位。八髎区是女性妇科反映点，可改善女性腰酸、腰凉等问题。八髎穴是调理女性妇科疾病和月经病的常用穴。您感觉力度可以吗？

第4步，双掌根推带脉4～5次分推回手排毒。带脉，主要有健脾利湿、调经止带的功效。

第5步，双手虎口来回推腰部肾区。腰部肾区属于膀胱经在腰部的循行部分，双手虎口来回推膀胱经有助于促进腰部经脉畅通、气血运行加快，缓解腰部疼痛、劳损，改善肾脏功能。

第6步，双手交替提拉带脉然后分推排毒。带脉，主要有健脾利湿，调经止带的功效。

第7步，搓热肾区及腰骶部安抚结束。搓热肾区和八髎区可改善肾脏功能，具有温肾补阳、强腰固肾、调理女性疾病的作用。

（2）腹部：

第1步，热敷。同腰部操作。

第2步，铺油，腰部安抚。同腰部操作。

第3步，顺时针打开通络油，点中脘穴、天枢穴、气海穴、关元穴、中极穴、子宫穴、归来穴，安抚施术区。点穴可以达到调动脏腑经脉经气，改善脏腑功能，调理肠胃功能、生殖功能、免疫功能，生理功能等。

第4步，双手掌交替顺任脉由巨阙穴至中极穴，顺双侧胃经由12肋骨游离缘至归来穴。中医认为，任主胞胎，任脉为阴脉之海，女子属阴，任脉对女性孕育生命、月经来潮都有着重要的作用。顺胃经有助于消化，增强胃蠕动，改善因消化功能低下或紊乱导致的胃胀、胃痛、胃酸等症。

第5步，掌心揉脐上、脐下、脐左、脐右及脐中。揉脐上能够促进肠胃蠕动，促进消化功能的改善，代表穴位如中脘穴；揉脐下可调理女性子宫，改善宫寒、月经不调，代表穴位如气海穴、关元穴、水道穴、归来穴等；揉脐左和脐右有助于促进肠蠕动，改善大肠功能失调引起的腹痛、腹泻、便秘等，代表穴位如天枢穴；揉脐中能够培本固元、温阳散寒，改善因中阳虚寒导致的畏寒怕冷，小便清长，遗尿，腹中寒，倦怠乏力等，代表穴位如神阙穴。

第6步，双手掌交替提拉带脉，双手分推反手排毒。带脉，主要有健脾利湿、调经止带的功效，主治痛经、月经不调、带下病、盆腔炎等，对腰部肥满松软有一定的调理作用。

第7步，双手拉抹带脉10次。

第8步，双手搓热暖子宫穴、神阙穴，灸法施灸于施术区30分钟。此手法对宫寒、痛经、月经不调、怕冷、畏寒、胃寒有调理作用。女士，冲任调理的手法已经做完，下面做艾灸疗法，艾灸具有补阳益气活血、抗炎、祛风除湿的多重功效，能迅速温通人体经络，祛除风寒湿等邪气，它和手法结合，可以起到事半功倍的效果。

3. 结束语　女士，冲脉、任脉、带脉调理项目到此就做完了，谢谢您的配合。如果你有什么意见和建议请告诉我们，我们一定积极改进。

六、注意事项

1）施术前注意房间光线和温度是否合适。

2）治疗时间约60分钟，手法施术时间以30分钟为宜，不宜太长；有心脏病史，腰腹部有手术史小于2年者，手法以轻柔为主，并询问患者感受，调整手法。

3）用毛巾包好非暴露部位，以防止药油弄脏衣服。

4）做艾灸时要随时观察温度，以免烫伤患者。温度以患者感觉舒适为度，不可过烫。

七、终末处理

1. **患者**　治疗结束为患者做治疗评价，针对患者情况给予简单的养生建议。流程结束嘱休息 5～10 分钟，喝温开水或养生药茶 1 杯。

2. **治疗车及物品整理**

1）治疗车清理干净，放于治疗室指定位置。

2）整理房间及床单元。

八、应急预案

1. **通络油过敏**　参照本章第一节"经筋推拿"处理方法。

2. **艾灸起疱**　参照本章第一节"经筋推拿"拔罐起疱处理方法。

九、知识储备

一级知识储备

1）中医的整体观念的理解，冲脉、任脉调理的重要性。

2）冲脉、任脉、带脉的循行路线、重点穴位的定位、主治功能。

3）肾俞穴、志室穴的定位、主治功能。

4）腹部重要穴位的定位、主治功能。

5）腰腹部疾患的症状和治疗的重要性。

6）冲脉和女性生殖系统的关系。

十、冲脉、任脉、带脉调理操作评分标准

冲脉、任脉、带脉调理操作评分标准见下表。

冲脉、任脉、带脉调理操作评分标准

项目总分 100 分	要　求	分值	评分说明	扣分
素质要求 5 分	仪表大方，举止端庄，态度和蔼，衣帽整齐，洗手，戴口罩	5	根据完成情况酌情扣分	

项目总分 100分		要　求	分值	评分说明	扣分
操作前准备 25分	告知	治疗所需时间、作用，操作方法，局部可能出现的症状等，取得患者合作	4	根据告知情况酌情扣分	
	评估	（四诊）现病史，既往史，家族史，过敏史，是否妊娠或月经期；施术部位皮肤情况、对疼痛的耐受度等	10	根据评估情况酌情扣分	
	物品	治疗车1辆。上层：取直径30厘米，深15～20厘米的器皿1个，加入10滴精油和温度60℃左右水1 500毫升；通络油（10～30毫升）1瓶，酒精灯、打火机各1个，艾条适量 下层：床单1条，毛巾（30厘米×70厘米）3条，浴巾1条，养生服1套	5	物品准备不完善酌情扣分	
	患者及环境	询问患者治疗前准备情况，取合理体位，松解衣物 室内整洁，保护隐私，注意保暖，避免对流风	6	两项各占3分，回答不完善可酌情扣分	
操作过程 40分	核对医嘱	核对姓名、诊断等	3	未核对扣3分；内容不全面酌情扣分	
	操作	按标准技术操作规程步骤操作（步骤附后，详写分值）	25	按表后详细分值评分	
	观察	治疗过程中询问患者感受：舒适度、疼痛情况；观察施术部位皮肤情况	7	未与患者沟通扣7分；内容不全面酌情扣分	
	治疗后	询问患者感受并告知相关注意事项；协助患者取舒适体位	5	未告知注意事项扣3分，未安置体位扣2分	
操作后 20分	整理	整理床单元，整理用物，物品清洗消毒并归位，洗手	5	整理不完善酌情扣分	
	评价	施灸部位准确，手法操作娴熟，与患者沟通良好，患者感觉达到预期目的	5	评价内容不完善酌情扣分	
	病历记录	详细病历记录治疗情况，签名	2	未记录扣2分；记录不完整扣1分	
	操作后处置	用物按《医疗机构消毒技术规范》处理	8	处置方法不正确，每项扣2分	
理论提问10分		冲脉、任脉、带脉调理的相关知识 冲任调理的操作注意事项	10	回答不全面每题扣2分；未答出每题扣5分	

总分：

主考老师签名：　　　　　　　　　　考核日期：　　　年　　月　　日

附　操作步骤及评分分值：

（1）腰部：

第1步，热敷。（1分）

第2步，铺油。（1分）

第3步，①打开通络油，点肾俞穴、志室穴，反手推八髎区，点按八髎穴，腰骶部安抚。②双手拇指点按以上穴位，然后转身向腰部双手拇指交替推八髎区，并点按八髎穴。（2分）

第4步，①双掌根推带脉4～5次，分推回手排毒。②双掌根交替从脊柱向外推一侧带脉然后换另外一侧。（2分）

第5步，双手虎口来回推腰部肾区。（2分）

第6步，双手交替提拉带脉然后分推排毒。（2分）

第7步，搓热肾区及腰骶部安抚，结束。（2分）

（2）腹部：

第1步，热敷。（1分）

第2步，铺油。（1分）

第3步，①顺时针打开通络油，点中脘穴、天枢穴、气海穴、关元穴、中极穴、子宫穴、归来穴，安抚施术区。②以一手中指或拇指为着力点，依次进行点按以上穴位。（2分）

第4步，双手掌交替顺任脉由巨阙穴至中极穴，顺双侧胃经由12肋骨游离缘至归来穴。（2分）

第5步，掌心按揉脐上、脐下、脐左、脐右及脐中。（2分）

第6步，双手掌交替提拉带脉，双手分推反手排毒。（2分）

第7步，双手拉抹带脉10次。（1分）

第8步，双手搓热暖子宫穴、神阙穴，根据患者具体情况进行腰部或腹部施灸30分钟。（2分）

第五节　五行悬灸

一、项目名称

五行悬灸项目是以传统中医灸法防病、治病养生保健理念为依托，配合天然植物精油，在任督二脉循经点穴，融合五行脐部给药技术，使用无烟艾条和悬灸器在腹部悬空施灸的疗法。

二、项目功能

疏通任督二脉，调和五脏阴阳，补益五脏虚损。

三、适应证

体质偏颇状态之气虚质、阳虚质、气郁质、痰湿质及肝、心、脾、肺、肾脏气不足等。

四、标准技术操作规程

1. 准备工作

（1）施术者操作前准备：施术者做好个人卫生（包括剪指甲），消毒洗手，衣帽整齐，戴口罩。

（2）物品准备：治疗车1辆。①上层。悬灸器1套；治疗盘1个，盘中纳入：五行悬灸精油1支，无烟艾条2支，酒精灯1个，打火机1个，脐疗药粉1份，专用脐贴1张。②下层。床单1条，毛巾（30厘米×70厘米）2条，浴巾1条，养生服1套。

（3）患者准备：换上养生服，取俯卧位于治疗床上，露出整个背部及腰骶部至八髎穴位置，上肢放于身体两侧。术者取一毛巾在背垂直方向压于裤腰边缘（毛巾1/4宽压于衣服内，以免五行悬灸精油弄脏衣服）。

2. 开始操作　无特殊说明，每个手法操作3遍。

（1）背部经络疏通（11分钟）：

第1步，铺油，背部安抚。①术者站于床头，取适量油在掌心处，双掌相对搓（以双手掌蘸满油但不滴下为度，不能滴到患者背部、头发及床单上），双掌分开放于脊柱两侧膀胱经由大椎穴水平开始，按照掌根→掌心→指部→指尖的次序充分贴于背部，然后按以上顺序抬离背部（除拇指外其余四指指尖不离开背部），再按照以上顺序重复贴于背部、抬离背部，直至腰骶部，使双掌经过的背部铺满油。②抬起双手，双掌指尖相对紧贴于背部放于脊柱两侧，由大椎穴水平向下平推至腰骶部，然后转掌与脊柱平行，回拉至大椎穴水平，双掌相离至肩部包肩，顺着斜方肌

的走行提拉至风池穴，中指点按风池穴。若患者背部面积较大，可重复以上动作1次，以背部铺满油但无多余油流动为度。（1分钟）

第2步，疏通督脉到八髎区。双手拇指相邻，于脊柱垂直方向放于督脉上，其余四指指尖向外贴于背部，拇指从大椎穴开始用力推督脉至八髎区（可直推也可分段推），推过后可背部安抚1～2遍。（1分钟）

第3步，拇指推夹脊穴。双手拇指直推双侧夹脊穴，也可分段推，有结节或条索的地方可重点疏通（拇指推或点按）。推至腰骶部，拇指交替弧形推八髎区。（2分钟）

第4步，拇指推膀胱经。操作同第3步，施术于膀胱经第一侧线。（2分钟）

第5步，双拳半握疏通膀胱经。双手半握拳以指间关节为着力点，分别疏通脊柱两侧膀胱经，有结节或条索的地方可重复推。（1分钟）

第6步，揉按肩井穴、天宗穴，疏通肩胛内侧线。拇指揉按肩井穴，拇指揉按天宗穴，拇指沿肩胛内侧线自上而下推。（1分钟）

第7步，腰部安抚，点腰部穴位，分推腰部。双手腰部安抚，双手拇指从上到下依次点腰椎一到腰椎四膀胱经穴位及腰骶部穴位。（2分钟）

第8步，搓热命门。双手重叠横搓腰部。（1分钟）

（2）腹部经络疏通（9分钟）：

第1步，铺油。把五行悬灸精油均匀地铺在患者腹部。（1分钟）

第2步，推任脉、胃经。双手交替推任脉，推双侧胃经（先左后右）。（2分钟）

第3步，点穴。用中指依次点按中脘穴、气海穴、关元穴、天枢穴。（2分钟）

第4步，掌根揉腹部。双手重叠用掌根依次由脐中、脐右、脐上、脐左、脐下揉按腹部。（2分钟）

第5步，拉抹带脉。双手虎口交替拉抹腹部。（2分钟）

（3）腹部施灸（40分钟）：

第1步，脐部给药。脐疗药粉将脐部填满，然后加入五行悬灸精油。

第2步，点燃无烟艾条。将无烟艾条一头点燃置于悬灸器内，盖上盖子。

第3步，悬灸。连接电源打开调速器。先把电源调速器与悬灸器连接，然后与电源连接。根据患者感受调节调速器，控制艾灸温度。

五、工作语言规范

1. **治疗前**　先生（女士）您好！欢迎您来到 ××，我是您的调理医师 ××，很高兴为您服务。今天做的项目是五行悬灸。此疗法运用天然植物精油，根据任督二脉的循经路线，结合推拿按摩技术，依据脐部给药原理，在脐部敷五脏调理药物，使用安全方便的无烟艾条悬灸器，进行悬灸，可温通经络、调和五脏气血、改善五脏功能。

治疗时间大概需要 60 分钟，您需要去洗手间吗？（不去）

先生（女士）房间温度和亮度可以吗？您需要把上衣脱掉，我帮您挂在衣架上。请您在这张床上取俯卧位。

2. **治疗中**　以下按步骤操作并配合语言艺术。

（1）背部：

您平时有哪里不舒服吗？我可以根据您的个人情况给予辨证调理。

第 1 步，铺油。五行悬灸精油是根据肝、心、脾、肺、肾不同功能特点而研制的个性化调理，针对性较强。

第 2 步，疏通督脉推八髎区。督脉为阳脉之海，疏通督脉能够激发和提升阳气，可改善阳虚引起的怕冷、手脚冰凉等。您感觉力度可以吗？

第 3 步，拇指推夹脊穴。夹脊穴与脏腑密切相关，是体内脏腑与背部体表相联通的点，解剖上每穴都有相应的椎骨下方发出的脊神经后支及其伴行的动脉、静脉分布，研究认为夹脊穴能调节自主神经的功能，故用夹脊穴治疗与自主神经功能有关的疾病，如血管性头痛、肢端感觉异常症、自主神经功能紊乱、脑血管病、高血压等。

第 4 步，拇指推膀胱经。

第 5 步，双拳半握疏通膀胱经。五脏六腑在膀胱经上都有一对对应背俞穴。背俞穴与脏腑有特殊的关系，在临床上能反映脏腑的虚实盛衰，当背俞穴出现各种异常反应，如结节、条索状物、压痛、丘疹等，往往能够反映相关脏腑的异常。我们通过辨证选取背俞穴调理，可以达到以局部调理整体的目的。膀胱经是人体的防御屏障，保护好膀胱经，激发其防御功能，能够提升正气，提高人体免疫力。

第 6 步，揉按肩井穴、天宗穴、肩胛内侧线。现代人伏案工作较多，肩颈部是最容易疲劳的地方，初期会有颈肩部疼痛，休息后缓解，如果长期不重视，就会逐渐形成颈椎病。通过专业中医手法进行肩颈部调理修复，可以有效地预防和治疗因颈椎病引起的肩背痛、手麻、头痛、头晕、失眠等。

第7步，腰部安抚，点腰部穴位，分推腰部。腰为肾之府。中医讲肾为先天之本，肾俞穴是肾脏精气输注于腰部的穴位，注重养肾，能够调理腰膝酸软、失眠健忘、神疲乏力，从而起到强腰补肾、增强男女生殖功能的作用。

（2）腹部经络疏通：

第1步，铺油。把五行悬灸精油均匀地涂在患者腹部。

第2步，推任脉，推胃经。任脉为阴脉之海，有调整人体阴经经气的作用，疏通胃经有利于调节胃肠消化功能。

第3步，点穴。点中脘穴、天枢穴有利于增强胃肠蠕动，促进消化；点气海穴、关元穴，有补气固元的作用。

第4步，掌根揉按腹部。双手重叠依次由脐中、脐左、脐上、脐右、脐下。揉按腹部，能够促进胃肠蠕动，增强消化功能，改善肠道功能失调引起的腹痛、便秘、腹泻等，代表穴位如中脘穴，天枢穴等。

第5步，拉抹带脉。带脉具有约束诸经、利湿健脾、调经止带的作用。有利于协调平衡各经络功能，调整脏腑功能。

（3）腹部施灸：

第1步，①脐部给药。脐部神阙穴当元神之门户，故有回阳救逆、开窍苏厥之功效。神阙穴位于腹之中部，人体之枢纽，又邻近胃、大肠、小肠和胞宫，此穴位能健脾胃、理肠止泻、益元固本、调养生理功能的作用。脐疗药粉、五行悬灸精油可以改善肝、心、脾、肺、肾五脏功能失常引起的各种病症，如肝木不达，肝郁出现的情绪抑郁、两胁胀痛、月经不调等；心气虚即"心气不足"引起的心悸、短气（活动时加剧）、胸闷不舒、自汗、脉细弱或结代等；脾气虚，脾阳虚引起的食少、腹胀、腹痛、便溏等；肺气虚引起的少气乏力，稍有劳作则气喘吁吁，呼吸气促；人体抗病能力低下等；肾阳虚引起的畏寒肢冷、神疲乏力、夜尿多等。

第2步，点燃无烟艾条。避免烟雾污染。

第3步，悬灸。可升高降低，根据不同体型，不同耐热程度、患者需求等可调至适宜高度，非常方便。

3.结束语　先生（女士），五行悬灸项目到此就做完了。感谢您积极的配合。如果您有什么意见和建议请告诉我们，我们一定积极改进。

六、注意事项

1）施术前注意房间光线和温度是否合适。

2）治疗时间约 60 分钟，手法施术时间以 20 分钟为宜，不宜太长；有心脏病史，脊柱椎体手术史小于 2 年者，手法以轻柔为主，并询问患者感受，调整手法。

3）女性患者长发者，注意用毛巾包好头发。

4）艾灸要随时观察温度，以免烫伤患者。温度以患者感觉舒适为度，不可过烫，告知患者并不是温度越高效果越好。

5）嘱患者 6 小时内不洗澡。

七、终末处理

1. 患者　治疗结束应把患者背部的油擦干净。嘱患者避免受凉，多饮温开水，当天不做剧烈运动。等患者整理好衣物后将其引领至休息处，嘱其休息 5 ～ 10 分钟，喝温开水或养生药茶 1 杯。

2. 治疗车及物品整理

1）治疗车清理干净，放于治疗室指定位置。

2）悬灸器及时整理，检查艾条燃烧情况，注意防火。

3）整理房间及床单元。

八、应急预案

1. 精油过敏　立即停用所用精油。过敏症状轻者以温水擦洗患处，重者给予抗过敏治疗。

2. 艾灸起疱　参照本章第一节"脊柱调理"拔罐起疱处理方法。

九、知识储备（与流程有关的知识点）

一级知识储备

1）中医的整体观念的理解，背部调理的重要性。

2）督脉的循行路线、重点穴位的定位、主治功能。

3）夹脊穴的定位、主治功能。

4）膀胱经的循行路线、背俞穴的定位和作用。

5）风池、风府、肩井、天宗穴的定位、归经、主治功能。

6）带脉的作用。

7）肾俞穴、命门穴命名的由来、定位、主治功能及其在整体调理中的重要性。

8）脐疗的作用。

9）五脏生理功能。

附　精油配方：

1）肝。荷荷巴油中加入迷迭香、佛手柑精油。

2）心。荷荷巴油中加入橙花精油。

3）脾。荷荷巴油中加入橙花、薄荷精油。

4）肺。荷荷巴油中加入茶树、尤加利精油。

5）肾。荷荷巴油中加入茴香精油。

十、五行悬灸操作评分标准

五行悬灸操作评分标准见下表。

五行悬灸操作评分标准

项目总分 100分		要　求	分值	评分说明	扣分
素质要求 5分		仪表大方，举止端庄，态度和蔼，衣帽整齐，洗手，戴口罩	5	根据完成情况酌情扣分	
操作前准备 25分	告知	治疗所需时间、作用，操作方法，局部可能出现的症状等，取得患者合作	4	根据告知情况酌情扣分	
	评估	（四诊）现病史，既往史，家族史，过敏史，是否妊娠或月经期；施术部位皮肤情况、对疼痛的耐受度等	10	根据评估情况酌情扣分	
	物品	治疗车1辆。上层：治疗盘1个，盘中放五行悬灸精油1支，无烟艾条2支，酒精灯1个，打火机1个，脐疗药粉1份，专用脐贴1张。悬灸器1套 下层：床单1条，毛巾（30厘米×70厘米）2条，浴巾1条，养生服1套	5	物品准备不完善酌情扣分	
	患者及环境	询问患者治疗前准备情况，取合理体位，松解衣物 室内整洁，保护隐私，注意保暖，避免对流风	6	两项各占3分，回答不完善可酌情扣分	

项目总分 100分		要　　求	分值	评分说明	扣分
操作过程 40分	核对医嘱	核对姓名、诊断等	3	未核对扣3分；内容不全面酌情扣分	
	操作	按标准技术操作规程步骤操作（步骤附后，详写分值）	25	按表后详细分值评分	
	观察	治疗过程中询问患者感受：舒适度、疼痛情况；观察施术部位皮肤情况	7	未与患者沟通扣7分；内容不全面酌情扣分	
	治疗后	询问患者感受并告知相关注意事项；协助患者取舒适体位	5	未告知注意事项扣3分，未安置体位扣2分	
操作后 20分	整理	整理床单元，整理用物，物品清洗消毒并归位，洗手	5	整理不完善酌情扣分	
	评价	施灸部位准确，手法操作娴熟，与患者沟通良好，患者感觉达到预期目的	5	评价内容不完善酌情扣分	
	病历记录	详细病历记录治疗情况，签名	2	未记录扣2分；记录不完全扣1分	
	操作后处置	用物按《医疗机构消毒技术规范》处理	8	处置方法不正确，每项扣2分	
理论提问10分		悬灸的相关知识 悬灸的操作注意事项	10	回答不全面每题扣2分；未答出每题扣5分	

总分：

主考老师签名：　　　　　　　　　考核日期：　　　　年　　月　　日

附　五行悬灸操作步骤及评分分值：

（1）背部经络疏通：

第1步，铺油。（1分）

第2步，疏通督脉到八髎区。（1.5分）

第3步，拇指推夹脊穴。（1.5分）

第4步，拇指推膀胱经。（1.5分）

第5步，双拳半握疏通膀胱经。（1.5分）

第6步，揉按肩井穴，天宗穴，疏通肩胛内侧线。（2分）

第7步，腰部安抚，点腰部穴位，分推腰部。（2分）

第8步，搓热命门。（1分）

（2）腹部经络疏通：

第1步，铺油。（1分）

第2步，推任脉、胃经。（2分）

第3步，点穴。（2分）

第4步，掌根揉按腹部。（2分）

第5步，拉抹带脉。（2分）

（3）腹部施灸：

第1步，脐部给药。（2分）

第2步，点燃无烟艾条。（1分）

第3步，连接电源打开调速器。（1分）

第六节　五体疏通

一、项目名称

"五体"一是指头、双上肢和双下肢，亦指筋、脉、肉、皮、骨。五体疏通是根据中医"整体观念"和经络的循行特点，重视头、双上肢，双下肢的经络和穴位对人体的调节作用，整合了头部经络疏通疗法，四肢肘膝关节以下经络疏通，足部反射区疗法的系统调理方法。

二、项目功能

疏通经络，调和气血，平衡阴阳，防病保健。

三、适应证

适用于头晕、失眠、易疲劳、肠胃功能紊乱、易手脚冰凉、头痛等亚健康状态的调理。

四、标准技术操作规程

1. 准备工作

(1)施术者操作前准备：施术者做好个人卫生（包括剪指甲），消毒洗手，衣帽整齐，戴口罩。

（2）物品准备：治疗车1辆。①上层。中药足浴水1桶，水深20～25厘米，通络油1瓶（10～30毫升），头部刮痧板1个。②下层。床单1条，毛巾（45厘米×75厘米）4条，浴巾1条，养生服1套。

（3）患者准备：嘱患者换上养生服，头发散下，饰品摘掉并收好。取坐位于治疗床上，双足试水温后进行足浴。

2. 开始操作　无特殊说明，每个手法操作3遍。

（1）头部操作（15分钟）：

头部按摩（8分钟，每步1分钟）：

第1步，点印堂，拉抹印堂穴至神庭穴。双手中指点按印堂穴，然后双手中指和无名指并齐交替从印堂穴向上拉抹至神庭穴。

第2步，抹眉弓至太阳穴并点按太阳穴，点睛明穴、攒竹穴、鱼腰穴、丝竹空穴，拉抹额头。双手拇指与其余四指分开，拇指指尖向下，拇指桡侧缘紧贴额头，从中间向两边抹眉弓至太阳穴，中指点按太阳穴，用双手拇指点按睛明穴、攒竹穴、鱼腰穴、丝竹空穴，双手拇指桡侧缘从额头中间向两边拉抹额头。

第3步，点按督脉、膀胱经，四指指腹按揉颞部，指关节按揉颞部至耳上角。双手拇指点头部督脉由神庭穴至百会穴，点头部膀胱经穴位由曲差穴至络却穴；双手四指指腹按揉颞部，四指关节按揉颞部至耳上角。

第4步，手扫头部胆经点率谷穴。四指自然屈曲，用指腹在侧头部来回扫头部胆经，同法操作右侧胆经，中指点按率谷穴。

第5步，点按听宫穴、听会穴，搓揉耳朵，点按翳风穴。双手中指点按听宫穴、听会穴，然后用双手食指和中指夹住耳朵根部做快速地上下往返搓揉耳朵至发热，然后中指点按翳风穴。

第6步，拿揉后颈部至大椎穴，点按风池穴、风府穴。一手置于头顶固定头部，另一手拇指与其余四指呈弓形，拿揉后颈部肌肉至大椎穴，然后拇指点按风池穴、风府穴。

第7步，拿揉斜方肌至上臂。用双手虎口拿揉斜方肌至上臂。

第8步，叩头部结束。双手立掌，掌心相对，指尖朝前，以小指掌指关节尺侧缘着力在头部进行有节律的叩击。

头部刮痧（7分钟）：

第1步，点百会穴，从百会穴向前刮至神庭穴。一手固定头部，另一手持刮痧

板，以刮痧板的一角为着力点点按百会穴，然后从百会穴向前刮至前发际神庭穴。（1分钟）

第2步，从百会穴放射状刮头部。用刮痧板从百会穴顺时针依次放射状刮头部。（2分钟）

第3步，刮前额。用刮痧板的一角刮拭前发际前、后1厘米范围，从左侧头维穴循序渐进刮至右侧头维穴，来回刮拭。（1分钟）

第4步，刮督脉、膀胱经、胆经。先左后右。刮痧板循经络刮督脉、膀胱经、胆经的头部循行，由前发际刮至后发际。先左后右。（2分钟）

第5步，梳理头部结束。用刮痧板的齿部将患者头发梳理整齐。（1分钟）

（2）上肢操作（主要操作肘关节以下部分，先左后右）（20分钟）：

第1步，拇指按揉肺经，点按尺泽穴、太渊穴。拇指揉法按揉肺经，由尺泽穴到太渊穴方向，拇指点按尺泽穴、太渊穴。

第2步，拇指按揉大肠经，点按阳溪穴、曲池穴。拇指揉法按揉大肠经，由阳溪穴到曲池穴方向，拇指点按阳池穴、曲池穴。

第3步，拇指按揉心包经，点按曲泽穴、内关穴。拇指揉法按揉心包经，由曲泽穴到内关穴方向，拇指点按曲泽穴、内关穴。

第4步，拇指按揉三焦经，点按外关穴、天井穴。拇指揉法按揉三焦经，由外关穴到天井穴方向，拇指点按外关穴、天井穴。

第5步，拇指按揉心经，点按少海穴、神门穴。拇指揉法按揉心经，由少海穴到神门穴方向，拇指点按少海穴、神门穴。

第6步，拇指按揉小肠经，点按阳谷穴、小海穴。拇指揉法按揉小肠经，由阳谷穴到小海穴方向，拇指点按阳谷穴、小海穴。

第7步，掌揉法按揉前臂，点腰痛点、落枕穴、合谷穴。

第8步，拇指推掌心，分推五指，搓揉掌根；拇指点按劳宫穴，叩掌，牵拉腕部。用拇指推掌心，拇指推法分推五指；术者一手固定患者腕部，一手与患者十指交叉，掌根搓揉患者掌根，然后用拇指点按劳宫穴，用手掌叩击患者手掌，牵拉患者腕部。

第9步，搓揉手指并牵拉指间关节。用拇指和食指搓揉患者手指，由拇指到小指依次搓揉，搓揉后牵拉指关节。

第10步，依次以揉法、拍法、抖法、牵拉法施术于上肢，结束。

足浴结束，用毛巾擦干双足，开始下肢操作。

（3）下肢操作（5分钟）：

第1步，双手五指揉髌骨。用双手五指指腹固定住髌骨，并做环形揉按髌骨。

第2步，按揉膝眼穴。双手拇指和食指分别按揉双膝的内外膝眼穴。

第3步，按揉足三里穴、三阴交穴。双手拇指按揉双侧足三里穴、三阴交穴。

第4步，双手拿揉小腿。双手拿揉小腿由内、外膝眼穴拿揉至解溪穴。

第5步，活动踝关节。双手握双足端，使双足依次左翻、右翻、背伸、跖屈。

第6步，空拳叩小腿外侧。双手空拳叩击小腿外侧。

（4）足部操作：操作顺序为足底→足内侧→足外侧→足背（先左后右），40分钟，左右各20分钟。

足底：左足先点心，看患者的心脏情况，并确定患者舒适的力度。

第1步，点肾上腺。肾上腺是点状穴，右手呈握拳状，拇指内收，用食指第二指间关节进行点按。

第2步，刮拭腹腔神经丛。腹腔神经丛是面状穴，右手呈握拳状，拇指内收，用食指第二指间关节进行左右两个半圆弧形刮拭。

第3步，点肾。肾是点状穴，右手呈握拳状，拇指内收，用食指第二指间关节进行点按。

第4步，刮拭输尿管。输尿管呈线状穴，右手呈握拳状，拇指内收，用食指第二指间关节从肾刮至膀胱位置，呈弧线进行刮拭。

第5步，点膀胱。呈点状穴，右手呈握拳状，拇指内收，用食指第二指间关节进行点按。

第6步，推尿道及会阴。尿道及会阴呈线状穴，右手拇指指腹由膀胱反射区向上弧形推。

第7步，刮拭前额（额窦）。前额（额窦）呈点状穴，左手拇指与其余四指固定在左脚的脚趾，右手空拳，用拇指指间关节进行横向刮拭。

第8步，推三叉神经。三叉神经呈线状穴，右手拇指由趾端向下直推。

第9步，点小脑及脑干。小脑及脑干呈点状穴，右手呈握拳状，拇指内收，用食指第二指间关节进行点按。

第10步，推颈项。颈项呈线状穴，用右手拇指指腹向内侧进行单向横推。

第11步，推鼻。鼻呈线状穴，用右手拇指指腹沿趾甲缘弧形推。

第12步，点大脑。大脑呈点状穴，右手呈握拳状，拇指内收，用食指第二指间关节进行点按。

第13步，点脑垂体。脑垂体呈点状穴，右手呈握拳状，拇指内收，用食指第二指间关节进行点按。

第14步，刮拭食管及气管。食管及气管呈线状穴，右手呈空拳，拇指内收，用食指第二指间关节向下进行单向刮拭。

第15步，刮拭甲状旁腺。甲状旁腺呈线状穴，右手呈空拳，拇指内收，用食指第二指间关节向下进行单向刮拭。

第16步，刮拭甲状腺。甲状腺呈线状穴，右手呈空拳，拇指内收，用食指第二指间关节向下进行单向刮拭。

第17步，刮拭其他趾额窦（头部）。其他趾额窦呈点状穴，左手拇指与其余四指固定在左脚的脚趾，右手空拳，用拇指指间关节进行横向刮拭。

第18步，点眼。眼呈点状穴，右手呈握拳状，拇指内收，用食指第二指间关节进行点按。

第19步，点耳。耳呈点状穴，右手呈握拳状，拇指内收，用食指第二指间关节进行点按。

第20步，刮拭斜方肌。斜方肌呈线状穴，右手呈空拳，拇指内收，用食指第一、第二指间关节面从外向内进行单向刮拭。

第21步，推肺及支气管。肺及支气管呈"人"字形穴，左右拇指相对，从足底两侧向足底进行推挤至中间部位，然后翻转拇指向上直推至足趾根部。

第22步，点心（右肝）。心呈点状穴，右手呈握空拳状，拇指内收，用食指第二指间关节进行点按。

第23步，点脾（右胆）。脾呈点状穴，右手呈握空拳状，拇指内收，用食指第二指间关节进行点按。

第24步，刮胃。胃呈面状穴，右手呈握空拳状，拇指内收，用食指第二指间关节向下进行单向直刮。

第25步，刮胰。胰呈面状穴，右手呈握空拳状，拇指内收，用食指第二指间关节向下进行单向直刮。

第26步，刮十二指肠。十二指肠呈面状穴，右手呈握空拳状，拇指内收，用食指第二指间关节向下进行单向直刮。

第27步，刮小肠。小肠呈面状穴，左手做固定，右手呈握拳状，拇指内收，用其余四指的第二指间关节向下进行单向直刮。

第28步，刮横结肠（右升结肠）。横结肠呈线状穴，用右手食指第二指间关节向外侧进行单向横刮至足底外侧缘。

第29步，刮降结肠（右横结肠）。降结肠呈线状穴，用右手食指第二指间关节向下进行单向竖刮拭至足跟部外上侧缘。

第30步，刮乙状结肠（右无）。乙状结肠呈线状穴，用右手食指第二指间关节向内侧进行单向横刮至足跟部内侧缘。

第31步，点失眠点。失眠点呈点状穴，右手呈握空拳状，拇指内收，用食指第二指间关节进行点按。

第32步，点生殖点。生殖点呈点状穴，右手呈握空拳状，拇指内收，用食指第二指间关节进行点按。

足内侧：

第1步，推颈椎。颈椎呈线状穴，用右手拇指指腹在内侧从前至后进行单向直推。

第2步，推胸椎。胸椎呈线状穴，用右手拇指指腹向内侧从前至后进行单向直推。

第3步，推腰椎。腰椎呈线状穴，用右手拇指指腹向内侧从前至后进行单向直推。

第4步，推骶骨。骶骨呈线状穴，用右手拇指指腹向内侧从前至后进行单向直推。

第5步，揉按子宫（前列腺）。子宫（前列腺）呈面状穴，用右手拇指指腹进行环形揉按。

第6步，推内侧直肠和肛门。内侧直肠及肛门呈线状穴，用右手拇指指腹从内侧脚踝向小腿内侧进行单向直推。

足外侧：

第1步，推肩。肩呈线状穴，用右手食指第二指间关节面从上向下进行单向直推。

第2步，点肘。肘呈线状穴位，用食指和中指的第二指间分别在肩的下方和膝的上方进行点按。

第3步，刮膝关节。膝关节呈线状穴位，用右手食指第二指间关节面从上而下进行弧形刮拭。

第4步，按揉卵巢（睾丸）。卵巢（睾丸）呈面状穴位，用拇指指腹进行环形揉按。

第5步，推肩胛骨。肩胛骨呈线状穴位，用两手拇指指腹上下并列从下向上进行单向直推。

第6步，推下腹部。下腹部呈线状穴位，用右手拇指腹从脚踝外侧向上进行单向直推至小腿外侧。

足背：

第1步，推上腭、下腭。用两手拇指平行，指尖相对，指腹相对横向推。

第2步，点扁桃体。用两手拇指指腹点按穴位。

第3步，点咽喉。用两手拇指指腹点按穴位。

第4步，揉按胸部和乳房。用两手拇指指腹做环形揉按。

第5步，推膈肌。用两手食指第二指间关节桡侧缘从中间向两边分推。

第6步，拇指点按解溪穴。

五、工作语言规范

1.*治疗前*　先生（女士）您好！我是您的调理医师，我叫××，很高兴为您服务。咱们今天做的是五体疏通项目。五体疏通项目主要是通过手法结合反射区疗法疏通头部、双上肢、双下肢的经络以达到平衡阴阳、调和气血、活血通络、防病保健的作用。对于因长期思虑过度、压力大、熬夜导致的失眠、头痛等，有很好的放松作用。

治疗时间大概需要80分钟，您需要去一下洗手间吗？（不去）

先生（女士），我们开始吧。请您换上养生服，我帮您把贵重物品存好，换上衣服之后背靠在沙发上。

2.*治疗中*　以下按步骤操作并配合语言艺术。

你平时哪里有不舒服吗？我可以根据您的个人情况给予辨证调理。

（1）头部按摩和头部刮痧：　现在为您做的是点百会穴。头为诸阳之会，百脉所通，对控制和调节人体的生命活动起着重要的作用。经穴按摩头部和刮痧，可以促进清阳上升，百脉调和，清醒头脑，增强记忆，您感觉力度可以吗？

（2）双上肢及下肢按摩：双上肢按摩主要是疏通手三阴和手三阳经脉。每条经脉上都分布着很多的穴位，如现在为您点按的穴位是尺泽穴，是肺经的穴位，能够调理肺脏的功能。心包经上的内关穴能够调节心脏的功能，通过疏通各经脉和点按重点穴位可改善肢体气血不通畅，达到防病保健的目的。双下肢主要是疏通足三阴经和足三阳经，其中足阳明胃经的足三里穴，有健脾和胃，强身健体，调和气血的作用。还有足太阴脾经的三阴交穴，是女性妇科常用穴，对女性常见病调理和保健都起着重要的作用。

（3）足部反射区按摩：中医学上认为，足三阴经和足三阳经分别起始和终止于足部，通过经络关系，共同维持着人体气血的运行。脏腑的病变可通过经络互相影响，疏通经络、调气血，又可达到治疗脏腑病变的效果。

3. 结束语　先生（女士），五体疏通项目已经做完了，您感觉怎么样？谢谢您的配合。如果您有什么意见和建议请告诉我们，我们一定积极改进。

六、注意事项

1）施术前注意房间光线和温度是否合适。

2）注意休息，不要熬夜，保持心情舒畅，及时添加衣服，注意保暖，避风寒。

3）保持精神愉悦，按时作息，治疗后6小时内不洗头、不洗澡。

七、终末处理

1. 患者　治疗结束后应把患者足部通络油擦干净。嘱患者避免受凉，多饮温开水，当天不做剧烈运动。等患者整理好衣物及随身物品后将其引领至大厅，嘱其休息5～10分钟，喝温开水或养生药茶1杯。

2. 治疗车及物品整理

1）治疗车清理干净，放于治疗室指定位置。

2）刮痧板清洗后，用酒精擦洗消毒，晾干后备用。

3）整理房间及床单元。

八、应急预案

通络油过敏参照本章第一节"经筋推拿"处理方法。

九、知识储备（与流程相关的知识点）

一级知识储备

1）五体的整体观念和重要性。

2）十二经络循行，重点头部及四肢肘膝关节以下的循行，及穴位的定位、主治功能。

3）足部反射区具体定位。

十、五体疏通操作评分标准

五体疏通操作评分标准见下表。

五体疏通操作评分标准

项目总分 100分		要　求	分值	评分说明	扣分
素质要求 5分		仪表大方，举止端庄，态度和蔼，衣帽整齐，洗手，戴口罩	5	根据完成情况酌情扣分	
操作前准备 25分	告知	治疗所需时间、作用，操作方法，局部可能出现的症状等，取得患者合作	4	根据告知情况酌情扣分	
	评估	（四诊）现病史，既往史，家族史，过敏史，是否妊娠或月经期；施术部位皮肤情况、对疼痛的耐受度等	10	根据评估情况酌情扣分	
	物品	治疗车1辆。上层：中药足浴水1桶，水深20～25厘米，通络油1瓶(10～30毫米)，头部刮痧板1个。下层：床单1条，毛巾（45厘米×75厘米）4条，浴巾1条，养生服1套	5	物品准备不完善酌情扣分	
	患者及环境	询问患者治疗前准备情况，取合理体位 室内整洁，保护隐私，注意保暖，避免对流风	6	体位选择、环境准备各3分，回答不完善酌情扣分	
操作过程 40分	核对医嘱	核对姓名、诊断等	3	未核对扣3分；内容不全面酌情扣分	
	操作	按标准技术操作规程步骤操作（步骤附后，详写分值）	25	按表后详细分值评分	
	观察	治疗过程中询问患者感受：舒适度、疼痛情况；观察施术部位皮肤情况	7	未与患者沟通扣7分；内容不全面酌情扣分	
	治疗后	询问患者感受并告知相关注意事项，协助患者取舒适体位	5	未告知注意事项扣3分，未安置体位扣2分	

项目总分 100分		要　　求	分值	评分说明	扣分
操作后 20分	整理	整理床单元，整理用物，物品清洗消毒并归位，洗手	5	整理不完善酌情扣分	
	评价	操作部位准确，手法操作娴熟，与患者沟通良好，患者感觉达到预期目的	5	评价内容不完善酌情扣分	
	病历记录	详细病历记录治疗情况，签名	2	未记录扣2分；记录不完全扣1分	
	操作后处置	用物按《医疗机构消毒技术规范》处理	8	处置方法不正确每项扣1分	
理论提问10分		五体疏通的相关知识 五体疏通的操作注意事项	10	回答不全面每题扣2分；未答出每题扣5分	

总分：

主考老师签名：　　　　　　　　考核日期：　　　年　　月　　日

附　操作步骤及评分分值：

（1）头部操作：

头部按摩（4分）：

第1步，点印堂，拉抹印堂穴至神庭穴。

第2步，抹眉弓至太阳穴并点按太阳穴，点睛明穴、攒竹穴、鱼腰穴、丝竹空穴，拉抹额头。

第3步，点按督脉、膀胱经，四指指腹按揉颞部，指关节按揉颞部至耳上角。

第4步，手扫头部胆经点率谷穴。

第5步，点按听宫穴、听会穴，搓揉耳朵，点按翳风穴。

第6步，拿揉后颈部至大椎穴，点按风池穴、风府穴。

第7步，拿揉斜方肌至上臂。用双手虎口拿揉斜方肌至上臂。

第8步，叩头部结束。

头部刮痧（3分）：

第1步，点百会穴，从百会穴向前刮至神庭穴。

第2步，从百会穴放射状刮头部。

第3步，刮前额。

第4步，刮督脉、膀胱经、胆经。先左后右。

第5步，梳理头部结束。

（2）上肢操作（5分）：

第1步，拇指按揉肺经，点按尺泽穴、太渊穴。

第2步，拇指按揉大肠经，点按阳溪穴、曲池穴。

第3步，拇指按揉心包经，点按曲泽穴、内关穴。

第4步，拇指按揉三焦经，点按外关穴、天井穴。

第5步，拇指按揉心经，点按少海穴、神门穴。

第6步，拇指按揉小肠经，点按阳谷穴、小海穴。

第7步，掌揉法按揉前臂，点腰痛点、落枕穴、合谷穴。

第8步，拇指推掌心，分推五指，搓揉掌根；拇指点按劳宫穴，叩掌，牵拉腕部。

第9步，搓揉手指并牵拉指间关节。

第10步，依次以揉法、拍法、抖法、牵拉法施术于上肢，结束。

（3）下肢操作（3分）：

第1步，双手五指揉髌骨。

第2步，按揉膝眼穴。

第3步，按揉足三里穴、三阴交穴。

第4步，双手拿揉小腿。

第5步，活动踝关节。

第6步，空拳叩小腿外侧。

（4）足部操作（共10分，左右各5分）：操作顺序为足底→足内侧→足外侧→足背（先左后右）。

足底：

第1步，点肾上腺。

第2步，刮拭腹腔神经丛。

第3步，点肾。

第4步，刮拭输尿管。

第5步，点膀胱。

第6步，推尿道及会阴。

第7步，刮拭前额（额窦）。

第8步，推三叉神经。

第9步，点小脑及脑干。

第10步，推颈项。

第11步，推鼻。

第12步，点大脑。

第13步，点脑垂体。

第14步，刮拭食管及气管。

第15步，刮拭甲状旁腺。

第16步，刮拭甲状腺。

第17步，刮拭其他趾额窦（头部）。

第18步，点眼。

第19步，点耳。

第20步，刮拭斜方肌。

第21步，推肺及支气管。

第22步，点心（右肝）。

第23步，点脾（右胆）。

第24步，刮胃。

第25步，刮胰。

第26步，刮十二指肠。

第27步，刮小肠。

第28步，刮横结肠（右升结肠）。

第29步，刮降结肠（右横结肠）。

第30步，乙状结肠（右无）。

第31步，点失眠点。

第32步，点生殖点。

足内侧：

第1步，推颈椎。

第2步，推胸椎。

第3步，推腰椎。

第4步，推骶骨。

第5步，揉按子宫（前列腺）。

第 6 步，推内侧直肠和肛门。

足外侧：

第 1 步，推肩。

第 2 步，点肘。

第 3 步，刮膝关节。

第 4 步，按揉卵巢（睾丸）。

第 5 步，推肩胛骨。

第 6 步，推下腹部。

足背：

第 1 步，推上腭、下腭。

第 2 步，点扁桃体。

第 3 步，点咽喉。

第 4 步，揉按胸部和乳房。

第 5 步，推膈肌。

第 6 步，拇指点按解溪穴。

第七节　药浴调理项目

一、项目名称

药浴调理项目运用中医传统手法与传统药浴相结合，加入芳香疗法，音乐疗法，融合视觉、触觉、嗅觉、听觉的良性刺激形成中医独特的全身经络的调理。

二、项目功能

疏通经络，畅行气血，蕴内达外，协调脏腑，提升活力。

三、适应证

免疫力低下、体寒、失眠、胃肠功能紊乱、焦虑、易疲劳等。

四、禁忌证

1）开放性损伤，局部伤口未愈合者，不宜进行此治疗，以防感染。

2）女性经期、孕期不宜进行药浴调理。

3）有高血压、心脏病等心脑血管疾病。心肺功能不全，体质虚弱的患者不宜进行此治疗，以防出现意外。

4）年老体弱及年幼的患者不宜进行此治疗，特殊情况需治疗，应有家属陪护，时间不宜过长。

5）对中药过敏者慎用此治疗，治疗过程中出现皮肤刺激症状者，应停止治疗及时请医师会诊。

6）空腹及饱餐后30分钟内不宜进行此治疗，空腹和饱餐后入浴容易造成眩晕疲劳。

7）高热大汗患者，不宜进行此治疗，以防虚脱。

五、标准技术操作规程

1. 准备工作

（1）施术者操作前准备：做好个人卫生（包括剪指甲），消毒洗手，衣帽整齐，戴口罩。

（2）物品准备：治疗车1辆。①上层。通络油（10～30毫升）1瓶，沐浴露1瓶，洗发水1瓶，香熏灯1个，音乐播放器1个，一次性药浴罩1个，美体膜1套，美体乳1支。②下层。浴帽1个，床单1条，浴巾2条，被子1条，毛巾（30厘米×70厘米）2条，一次性内裤2条，养生服1套。

（3）患者准备：嘱患者更衣，沐浴，注意脚下，防止滑倒。

2. 开始操作

（1）泡浴（40分钟）：

第1步，准备泡浴水，打开音乐、香熏灯，备好茶饮。

第2步，在浴桶内，铺一次性药浴罩，加适量水（视患者具体情况而定，一般加水至药浴桶的1／2～2／3），放入药液（成人配方适量，儿童酌减，水温37～40℃，以38℃为最佳）（附药方：益气消疲方、舒肩解痉方、暖宫散寒方、舒肝解郁方、养心安神方等）。

第3步，调好水温后，嘱患者进行泡浴。随时询问患者泡浴情况，若有不适，立即停止泡浴并依具体情况进行相应处理。

（2）背部按摩（10分钟）：每个步骤2遍。

第1步，铺油，背部安抚。①术者站于床头，取适量通络油在掌心处，双掌相对搓（以双手掌蘸满油但不滴下为度，不能滴到患者背部、头发及床单上），双掌分开放于脊柱两侧膀胱经由大椎穴水平开始，按照掌根→掌心→指部→指尖的次序充分贴于背部，然后按以上顺序抬离背部（除拇指外其余四指指尖不离开背部），再按照以上顺序重复贴于背部、抬离背部，直至腰骶部，使双掌经过的背部铺满油。②抬起双手，双掌指尖相对紧贴于背部放于脊柱两侧，由大椎穴水平向下平推至腰骶部，然后转掌与脊柱平行，回拉至大椎穴水平，双掌相离至肩部包肩，顺着斜方肌的走行提拉至风池穴，中指点按风池穴。

第2步，疏通督脉，双手重叠搓热督脉。双手拇指相邻与脊柱垂直方向放于督脉上，其余四指指尖向外贴于背部，拇指从大椎穴开始均匀用力推督脉至腰骶部八髎区，左手叠放至右手之上从大椎穴至八髎区搓热督脉。

第3步，推膀胱经返手拉回至手指尖排毒。双手拇指直推双侧膀胱经第一线也可分段推，其余四指指尖向外贴于背部至腰骶部，除拇指外其余四指掌面并拢外贴两侧背部返手过肩膀，顺手臂推至指尖排毒。

第4步，疏通两胁部。沿身体两侧（腋下至12肋骨游离缘）用双手拇指食指顺肋骨走向交替推。

第5步，双手拇指点大椎穴及背部膀胱经第一侧线上穴位。

第6步，太极式推背。双手交替画圆推整个背部。

第7步，双手拇指点按命门穴。

（3）臀部按摩（5分钟）：每个步骤2遍。

第1步，铺油。双手呈扇形铺开通络油。

第2步，点穴。拇指点按环跳穴、承扶穴。

第3步，提臀部。双手推揉臀部侧面向上提拉。

第4步，双手拇指点环跳穴、承扶穴。背部安抚，结束。

（4）腿后侧按摩（5分钟）：每个步骤2遍。

第1步，铺油。双手交替直线铺开通络油。

第2步，点按承扶穴、委中穴、承山穴。

第3步，双手疏通腿后面膀胱经。

第4步，点承扶穴、委中穴、承山穴，拿揉小腿部肌肉。

（5）胸部按摩（5分钟）：注意查找结节，每个步骤2遍。

第1步，铺油。

第2步，点按天突穴、膻中穴、乳根穴、屋翳穴、云门穴。

第3步，提升乳房。四指并拢双手交替由外侧向内提拉。

第4步，查找结节。四指指腹轻轻局部揉按乳房，如有结节根据情况嘱患者进一步检查。

第5步，点按天突穴、膻中穴、乳根穴、屋翳穴、云门等穴。

（6）腹部按摩（5分钟）：每个步骤2遍。

第1步，铺油。

第2步，点按上脘穴、中脘穴、下脘穴、气海穴、关元穴等。

第3步，疏通任脉。双手掌根从上脘穴向下推任脉到中极穴。

第4步，疏通侧腰部。从侧腰沿髂骨最高点上缘拉至中极穴结束，返手做另一侧。

第5步，双手推揉侧腰部。

第6步，双手搓热敷神阙穴。

第7步，排毒。双手掌根相对分推至侧腰部，然后从腰部拉回排毒。

（7）手臂按摩（5分钟）：每个步骤2遍。

第1步，铺油。

第2步，点按曲池穴、手三里穴、合谷穴、劳宫穴等。

第3步，搓揉手臂。

第4步，放松手臂。

第5步，提拉手臂。

（8）腿前侧按摩（5分钟）：每个步骤2遍。

第1步，铺油。

第2步，点按风市穴、血海穴、梁丘穴、足三里穴、阴陵泉穴、三阴交穴等。

第3步，双手掌面向下推阳明胃经循行线返手向上推脾经。

（9）淋浴及美体护理（40分钟）：

第1步，按要求进行淋浴清洁。

第2步，敷美体膜（不包括头面部和足部）。裹上保鲜膜，停留20分钟。

第3步，卸下美体膜。

第4步，涂上美体乳。

六、工作语言规范

1. **治疗前**　先生（女士）您好！欢迎您来到××，我是您的调理医师××，很高兴为您服务！咱们今天做的是药浴调理项目，药浴中的药物成分快速透过皮肤、孔窍和穴位进入体内，借助热力作用于全身肌表，循经络血脉，内达脏腑，由表及里，融合循经推法、运法可以起到疏通经络、调整阴阳、协调脏腑、运行气血、濡养全身的作用。

先生（女士），治疗时间大概需要120分钟，您需要去洗手间吗？（不去）

您感觉房间光线和温度是否合适？（可以）

请您先更衣和沐浴，药浴水温已调好。

2. **治疗中**　以下按步骤操作并配合语言艺术。

您平时哪里有不舒服吗？我可以根据您的个人情况给予辨证调养。

（1）泡浴：先生（女士）您感觉水温可以吗？（很好）。泡浴时间20分钟，如有不适，随时呼叫我们。

先生（女士），现在开始给您做全身按摩，按摩是根据中医的经络穴位来进行循经点穴，在治疗过程中，请您感觉一下力度如何，如有不适，请及时告知。

（2）背部按摩：督脉为阳脉之海，疏通督脉可提升阳气，预防和改善阳虚怕冷，手脚冰凉等。五脏六腑在膀胱经上都有一对相对应的背俞穴，背俞穴的异常反应能反映脏腑的虚实盛衰，通过辨证调理局部以达到整体调理的效果，膀胱经也是人体的防御屏障，增强其功能有利于防御风、寒、暑、湿、燥，火等，有效提高人体正气，增强免疫力。疏通肩、颈、腰、背，可改善因肩颈腰背部劳损引起的各种不适症状。

（3）臀部按摩：可通血脉，改善臀部的血液循环。

（4）腿后侧按摩：促进腿部血液循环，缓解肌肉疲劳等。

（5）胸部按摩：根据中医经络的关系，乳头属肝，乳房属胃。久病体虚、劳累过度或平时饮食不规律，会损伤脾胃而致气血生化无源，使乳房营养乏源。平时常按摩膻中穴、乳根穴、足三里穴有助于刺激肝胃经脉，能疏肝补血，养护乳房气血。气血充足方可改善乏力、食欲不振、腹胀、头晕、眼花、面色苍白等气血虚弱的现象。常按摩内关穴、膈俞穴、肝俞穴等，可改善两胁胀痛、心情抑郁、乳房胀痛等肝气郁滞的症状。

（6）腹部按摩：通过揉按腹部经络、穴位促进胃肠蠕动功能，利于排除糟粕及浊气，对于胃肠功能不好引起的便秘、腹胀，任脉不通引起的小腹坠胀、凉痛起到很好的调理作用。而且经常按摩腹部增强腹部脂肪代谢，有减肥功效。

（7）手臂按摩：可增强局部血液循环，缓解手臂肌肉疼痛等。

（8）腿前侧按摩：四肢部循经推拿和穴位点按，可以调整脏腑功能，同时可以疏通经络，促进局部的血液循环，有效增强肌肉力量和关节韧带柔韧性，使四肢协调能力增强，也有利于脂肪燃烧，起到减肥的作用。

操作过程中或操作后如有排气、小便增多，属正常现象。

3. 结束语　先生（女士），药浴调理项目已经做完了。感谢您的积极配合，如果您有什么意见或建议，请告诉我们，我们一定积极改进。本项目建议每周做1次，希望下次再见。

七、注意事项

1）泡浴水温以38℃为佳。

2）操作期间注意房间温度，以防患者受凉。

八、终末处理

1. 患者　治疗结束后嘱患者避免受凉，多饮温开水，当天不做剧烈活动。患者整理好衣服及随身物品后引领至休息处，嘱其休息5～10分钟，喝温开水或养生茶1杯。

2. 治疗车及物品整理

1）治疗车清理干净，放于治疗室指定位置。

2）整理房间及床单元。

3）患者离开后，将水放出，消毒药浴桶，擦拭残留消毒液，晾干后备用。

九、应急预案

1. 药浴过敏　立即停用所用药液，过敏症状轻者以温水冲洗患处，重者给予抗过敏治疗。

2. 药浴晕厥　若有头昏、恶心等症状，立即让患者出浴，平卧，给予葡萄糖液或生理盐水适量口服，开窗通风待患者稳定，如果不能缓解，立即就医。

十、知识储备（与流程有关的知识点）

1. 一级知识储备

1）中医的整体观念的理解，中药沐浴调理的重要性。

2）膀胱经的作用。

3）带脉的作用。

4）芳香疗法及药物泡浴的原理和作用。

5）音乐疗法的作用。

2. 附方

附方 1　益气消疲方（黄芪建中汤）：

黄芪、桂枝、白芍、生姜、大枣、炙甘草、党参。

附方 2　舒肩解痉方（身痛逐瘀汤）：

桃仁、当归、川芎、秦艽、甘草、延胡索、羌活、没药、香附、牛膝。

附方 3　暖宫散寒方（艾附暖宫丸）：

艾叶、香附、吴茱萸、肉桂、当归、川芎、白芍、地黄、黄芪、续断。

附方 4　舒肝解郁方（柴胡疏肝散）：

柴胡、白芍、枳实、甘草、陈皮、香附、川芎。

附方 5　养心安神方：

归脾汤（用于气血不足证）：党参、白术、黄芪、当归、甘草、茯神、远志、酸枣仁、木香、龙眼肉、生姜、大枣。

酸枣仁汤（用于阴血不足证）：川芎、知母、茯神、甘草、酸枣仁。

十一、药浴操作评分标准

药浴操作评分标准见下表。

药浴操作评分标准

项目总分 100分	要　求	分值	评分说明	扣分
素质要求 5分	仪表大方，举止端庄，态度和蔼，衣帽整齐，洗手，戴口罩	5	根据完成情况酌情扣分	

项目总分 100 分		要　求	分值	评分说明	扣分
操作前准备 25 分	告知	治疗所需时间、作用，操作方法，局部可能出现的症状等，取得患者合作	4	根据告知情况酌情扣分	
	评估	（四诊）现病史，既往史，家族史，过敏史，是否妊娠或月经期；施术部位皮肤情况、对疼痛的耐受度等	10	根据评估情况酌情扣分	
	物品	治疗车 1 辆。上层：通络油（10～30 毫升）1 瓶，沐浴露 1 瓶，洗发水 1 瓶，香熏灯 1 个，音乐播放器 1 个，一次性药浴罩 1 个，美体膜 1 套，美体乳 1 支 下层：浴帽 1 个，床单 1 条，浴巾 2 条，被子 1 条，毛巾（30 厘米 ×70 厘米）2 条，一次性内裤 2 条，养生服 1 套	5	物品准备不完善酌情扣分	
	患者及环境	询问患者治疗前准备情况，取合理体位，松解衣物 室内整洁，保护隐私，注意保暖，避免对流风	6	体位选择、环境准备各 3 分，回答不完善可酌情扣分	
操作过程 40 分	核对医嘱	核对姓名、诊断等	3	未核对扣 3 分；内容不全面酌情扣分	
	操作	以标准技术操作规程步骤操作（步骤附后，详写分值）	25	按表后详细分值评分	
	观察	治疗过程中询问患者感受：舒适度、疼痛情况；观察施术部位皮肤情况	7	未与患者沟通扣 7 分；内容不全面酌情扣分	
	治疗后	询问患者感受并告知相关注意事项；协助患者取舒适体位	5	未告知注意事项扣 3 分，未安置体位扣 2 分	
操作后 20 分	整理	整理床单元，整理用物，物品清洗消毒并归位，洗手	5	整理不完善酌情扣分	
	评价	操作部位准确，手法操作娴熟，与患者沟通良好，患者感觉达到预期目的	5	评价内容不完善酌情扣分	
	病历记录	详细病历记录治疗情况，签名	2	未记录扣 2 分；记录不完全扣 1 分	
	操作后处置	用物按《医疗机构消毒技术规范》处理	8	处置方法不正确，每项扣 1 分	
理论提问 10 分		药浴的相关知识 药浴的操作注意事项	10	未答出每题扣 5 分；回答不全面每题扣 2 分	

总分：

主考老师签名：　　　　　　　　考核日期：　　　年　　月　　日

附　操作步骤及评分分值：

（1）泡浴（3分）：泡浴时间20分钟。

（2）背部按摩（5分）：

第1步，铺油。

第2步，疏通督脉，双手重叠搓热督脉。

第3步，推膀胱经返手拉回至手指尖排毒。

第4步，疏通两胁部。

第5步，双手拇指点大椎穴及背部膀胱经第一侧线上穴位。

第6步，太极式推背。

第7步，双手拇指点按命门穴。

（3）臀部按摩（2分）：

第1步，铺油。

第2步，点穴。

第3步，提臀部。

第4步，双手拇指点环跳穴、承扶穴。

（4）腿后部按摩（2分）：

第1步，铺油。

第2步，点按承扶穴、委中穴、承山穴。

第3步，双手疏通腿后面膀胱经。

第4步，点承扶穴、委中穴、承山穴，拿揉小腿部肌肉。

（5）胸部按摩（4分）：

第1步，铺油。

第2步。点按天突穴、膻中穴、乳根穴、屋翳穴、云门穴。

第3步，提升乳房。

第4步，查找结节。

第5步，点按天突穴、膻中穴、乳根穴、屋翳穴、云门穴等。

（6）腹部按摩（4分）：

第1步，铺油。

第2步，点按上脘穴、中脘穴、下脘穴、气海穴、关元穴等。

第3步，疏通任脉。

第4步，疏通侧腰部。

第5步，双手推揉侧腰部。

第6步，双手搓热敷神阙穴。

第7步，排毒。

（7）手臂按摩（3分）：

第1步，铺油。

第2步，点按曲池穴、手三里穴、合谷穴、劳宫穴等。

第3步，搓揉手臂。

第4步，放松手臂。

第5步，提拉手臂。

（8）腿前侧按摩（2分）：

第1步，铺油。

第2步，点按风市穴、血海穴、梁丘穴、足三里穴、阴陵泉穴、三阴交穴等。

第3步，双手掌面向下推阳明胃经循行线返手向上推脾经。

第八节　督灸

一、项目名称

督灸是在督脉的颈、胸、腰脊椎上施以"隔物灸"，从而达到防病治病，强身健体的一种中医外治法。

二、项目功能

益肾通督，温阳散寒，壮骨透肌，破瘀散结，通痹止痛。

三、适应证

1）适用于缓解因风寒、邪湿所致的颈、肩、腰、腿等关节疼痛及软组织扭挫伤所致的疼痛。

2）适用于畏寒性疾病，如手脚冰凉、宫寒痛经等。

3）适用于气虚所致疾病，慢性疲劳综合征、免疫力低下等。

四、禁忌证

1）有严重内科疾病者、装有心脏起搏器者、代偿不全的心脏病患者禁用。高热患者、糖尿病患者禁用。

2）有出血倾向性疾病者、局部皮肤破损及感染者、体质高度过敏者禁用。

3）女性经期、孕期不用。

4）急性损伤不用。

5）儿童必须在成人的监护下使用。

五、标准技术操作规程

1. 准备工作

（1）施术者操作前准备：施术者做好个人卫生（包括剪指甲），消毒双手，衣帽整齐，戴口罩。

附1　姜丝的制作：生姜适量（普通生姜经处理后出丝率约为55%），将生姜切成小块状，装入料理机，接通电源，将生姜打碎成泥状，在打泥过程中可以轻轻摇动料理机，这样可以加速打姜泥的过程。取出打好的姜泥，用双手均匀挤压，将姜汁挤出，达到轻度施压时无姜汁流出为宜。

附2　艾炷的制作：艾绒100克，将其分为五等份，把每一份艾绒放在一手的掌心内，用另一手向其对抗施压互捻，捻成椭圆状或长条状，长度约为5厘米，越结实越好，放置时不散落艾绒为宜。

（2）物品准备：治疗车1辆。①上层：取一大小合适器皿盛备好的姜泥700克（女士）、800克（男士），75%酒精棉球，艾炷5个，酒精灯1个，打火机1个，线香1根，督灸器1个。②下层：床单1条，毛巾（30厘米×70厘米）2条，浴巾1条，养生服1套。③督灸器具尽量选用实木材质，其隔热性较为稳定，具体选择尺寸可参考下图。

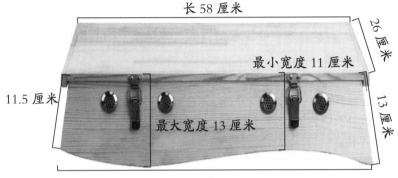

（3）患者准备：嘱患者换上养生服，取俯卧位于治疗床上，露出背部大椎穴至八髎穴位置，上肢放于身体两侧。

2. 开始操作

第1步，消毒。以75%酒精棉球自上而下沿脊柱常规消毒3遍。（3分钟）

第2步，放置艾炷。将5个艾炷置于督灸器里上下依次摆开。（2分钟）

第3步，定位。将督灸器置于大椎穴至八髎穴的脊柱部位。（1分钟）

第4步，点火。依次用线香自下而上点燃艾炷两端。（3分钟）

第5步，控温。施灸开始后进行计时。约20分钟要询问患者温度感觉如何（通常在20分钟的时候温度会达到最高点），有无烫感。如患者感到烫感明显，立即将督灸器取下，放置在干净的位置并迅速将消过毒的毛巾铺在有烫感的部位，然后重新将灸盒放置好。5分钟左右，再次询问患者感觉。艾灸时间约35分钟时，询问患者温度。诉温度稍降，即可将毛巾取下，继续灸10分钟即可结束本次灸疗。（50分钟）

第6步，操作结束取下督灸器，并清洁患者背部汗液及姜汁。（1分钟）

六、工作语言规范

1. 治疗前　先生（女士）您好！欢迎您来到××，我是您的调理医师××，很高兴为您服务。咱们今天做的是督灸项目。督灸具有益肾通督、温阳散寒、壮骨透肌、破瘀散结、通痹止痛的功效。

治疗时间大概需要60分钟，您需要去一下洗手间吗？（不去）

先生（女士），请您把上衣脱掉，我帮您挂在衣架上。您在这张床上取俯卧位。

2. 治疗中　以下按步骤操作并配合语言艺术。

第1步,消毒。先生（女士）您好！根据您的治疗需要,我现在对您的施灸部位进行消毒,因使用的是酒精,会稍微有些刺激皮肤,您稍微忍耐下。

第2步,放置督灸盒。

第3步,定位。先生（女士）我给您灸的是督脉的背部穴位,督脉与任脉、冲脉三者同起于胞中,督脉行于腰背部,任脉、冲脉行于腹胸部；督脉为阳脉之海,总督人身诸阳,诸阴经通过经别的联系合于阳经,因此认为督脉可以沟通全身经络,通过督灸的综合作用激发协调诸经,发挥经络内连脏腑、外络肢节、沟通内外、运行气血、平衡阴阳的功效,从而达到养生保健的目的。对于没有疾病的人可起到保健与养生的作用。现代社会由于人们长期工作劳累,熬夜,饮食上吃太多寒凉食物（如冰箱里冷冻的食物）,还有冷气的过度使用,这些都消耗了人体的阳气。人们感到身体越来越疲惫,精神越来越消沉,这些都是人们常说的"亚健康"状态。这些症状现代医学目前无特效方法。但是通过督灸这种物理性的治疗干预方法不仅可以起到改善症状的作用,还可以起到预防与保健的作用,这也是现代社会所提倡的"治未病"的保健养生思想。

第4步,点火。依次用线香自下而上点燃艾炷两端。先生（女士）现在已把艾炷点着,温度会慢慢上升,感觉烫或有其他不适,请及时与我沟通。

3.结束语　先生（女士）,督灸项目治疗已结束了,谢谢您积极的配合。如果有什么建议请告诉我们,我们积极改进。

七、注意事项

1）治疗期间注意房间温度及患者保暖。

2）灸疗期间要随时观察温度,以免烫伤患者,温度以患者感觉舒适为度,不可过烫。

3）老年患者不宜俯卧位太长时间,可适当缩短治疗时间。

4）嘱患者治疗后6小时内不洗澡。

八、终末处理

1.患者　治疗结束后应把患者背部的汗液及姜汁擦干净。嘱患者避免受凉,饮温开水,当天不做剧烈运动。等患者整理好衣物后将其引领至大厅,嘱其休息5～10分钟,喝温开水或养生药茶1杯。

2.治疗车及物品整理

1）治疗车清理干净，各物品归位，治疗车放于治疗室指定位置。

2）督灸器内、外清洁干净，晾干备用。

3）整理房间及床单元。

九、应急预案

1. 头晕　治疗结束后，有少数患者会出现头晕现象，是由于体位突然改变所引起，给予葡萄糖液适量口服，平卧稍作休息即可恢复。若不缓解给予对应处理，必要时请上级医师给予指导。

2. 灸疗起疱　参考本章第一节"脊柱调理"拔罐处理方法。

十、知识储备（与流程有关的知识点）

一级知识储备

1）中医的整体观念的理解，背部调理的重要性。

2）督脉的循行路线、重点穴位的定位、主治功能。

3）夹脊穴的定位、主治功能。

4）阴阳学说的基本内容及其在中医学中的应用。

十一、督灸操作评分标准

督灸操作评分标准见下表。

督灸操作评分标准

项目总分 100分	要　求	分值	评分说明	扣分
素质要求 5分	仪表大方，举止端庄，态度和蔼，衣帽整齐，洗手，戴口罩	5	根据完成情况酌情扣分	

项目总分 100分		要　求	分值	评分说明	扣分
操作前准备 25分	告知	治疗所需时间、作用，操作方法，局部可能出现的症状等，取得患者合作	4	根据告知情况酌情扣分	
	评估	（四诊）现病史，既往史，家族史，过敏史，是否妊娠或月经期；施术部位皮肤情况、对疼痛的耐受度等	10	根据评估情况酌情扣分	
	物品	治疗车1辆。上层：器皿1个，姜泥700克（女士）、800克（男士），75%酒精棉球，艾炷5个，酒精灯1个，打火机1个，线香1根，督灸器1个 下层：床单1条，毛巾（30厘米×70厘米）2条，浴巾1条，养生服1套，督灸器1个	5	物品准备不完善酌情扣分	
	患者及环境	询问患者治疗前准备情况，取合理体位，松解衣物 室内整洁，保护隐私，注意保暖，避免对流风	6	两项各占3分，回答不完善可酌情扣分	
操作过程 40分	核对医嘱	核对姓名、诊断等	3	未核对扣3分；内容不全面酌情扣分	
	操作	按标准技术操作规程步骤操作（步骤附后，详写分值）	25	按表后详细分值评分	
	观察	治疗过程中询问患者感受：舒适度、疼痛情况；观察施术部位皮肤情况	7	未与患者沟通扣7分；内容不全面酌情扣分	
	治疗后	询问患者感受并告知相关注意事项；协助患者取舒适体位	5	未告知注意事项扣3分，未安置体位扣2分	
操作后 20分	整理	整理床单元，整理用物，物品清洗消毒并归位，洗手	5	整理不完善酌情扣分	
	评价	操作部位准确，手法操作娴熟，与患者沟通良好，患者感觉达到预期目的	5	评价内容不完善酌情扣分	
	病历记录	详细病历记录治疗情况，签名	2	未记录扣2分；记录不完全扣1分	
	操作后处置	用物按《医疗机构消毒技术规范》处理	8	处置方法不正确每项扣2分	
理论提问10分		督灸的作用 督灸的操作注意事项	10	回答不全面每题扣2分；未答出每题扣5分	

总分：

主考老师签名：　　　　　　考核日期：　　　年　　月　　日

附 操作步骤及评分分值：

第1步，消毒。（4分）

第2步，放置艾炷。（4分）

第3步，定位。（4分）

第4步，点火。（4分）

第5步，控温。（7分）

第6步，操作结束取下督灸器，并清洁患者背部汗液及姜汁。（2分）

Proper Technical Operation Specifications of TCM Health Preservation

Chapter One
Basic Theory of Chinese Medicine

Section 1   The Theory of Viscera

Viscera is a collective term of the internal organs of human body, including the five zang-organs, six fu-organs and extraordinary fu-organs. The five zang-organs include the liver, heart, spleen, lung and kidney; the six fu-organs include the gallbladder, stomach, small intestine, large intestine, bladder, triple energizer; and the extraordinary fu-organs include the brain, marrow, bone, vessel, gallbladder and uterus. The functions of the zang-organs and fu-organs are different.The physiological function of the five zang-organs is to transform and store essence, qi, blood and body fluid; while that of the six fu-organs is to receive, decompose water and food, transport and transform and excrete the waste. The extraordinary fu-organs, differing from the five zang-organs and six fu-organs, are similar to the six fu-organs in morphology of being hollow inside with a cavity and to the zang-organs in function of storing essence. Therefore they are known as the extraordinary fu-organs. The gallbladder also belongs to one of the six fu-organs and is introduced in the section of "six fu-organs". The uterus is also introduced after the section of "six fu-organs". Others like brain, marrow, bone and vessels belong to five zang-organs and are described in the sections of "kidney" and "heart".

The viscera are an organic whole. There is close relationship between zang-organs, between fu-organs as well as between zang-organs and fu-organs. Besides, there is inseparable relationship between the viscera and body tissues (tendons, vessels, muscles, skin, bone) and external organs (nose, mouth, tongue, eyes, ears, anus and urethra). Qi, blood, and body fluid are indispensable substances for maintaining the life activities of the human body. Their production, circulation and distribution must be completed through different visceral functions. Qi, blood and body fluid are the material basis for the various functions of the viscera. Therefore, they are closely related between the viscera, between the viscera and qi, blood and body fluid in physiological functions and pathological changes.

The concept of viscera in Chinese medicine is not exactly the same as that in western medicine. The function of one organ in Chinese medicine may include that of several organs in western medicine; the function of one organ in western medicine may be involved in that of several organs in Chinese medicine. This is due to the fact that the viscera in Chinese medicine is not only an anatomical concept, but more importantly a physiological or pathological concept. For example, in addition to representing an anatomical entity, the "heart" in the viscera also includes the function of spirit and thinking activities. Therefore, the functions of the viscera in Chinese medicine cannot be equated with those of the organs in western medicine.

The Five Zang-organs

1. The liver

The liver is located in the abdomen, below the diaphragm and in the right rib-side. Its main function is to govern shuxie (dredging and regulating) and to store blood.

1.1 To dredge and regulate

Shuxie in Chinese means to dredge and smooth the route of something. The liver governing shuxie means that the liver has the function of smoothing the movement of qi. The function of dredging and regulating is mainly demonstrated in two aspects:

1.1.1 Emotional aspect

The liver has the function of regulating emotional activities. The mental and emotional activities are dominated by the heart and closely related to the liver. Only when the liver's function of dredging and regulating is normal and qi movement is smooth, can qi and blood flow harmoniously and people enjoy happiness and pleasure. If qi activity is in disorder due to failure of the liver to dredge and regulate, it will lead to abnormal changes of mental activities, such as chest and hypochondriac distension, melancholy, sentimentality due to stagnation of liver qi. If liver qi is hyperactive, it will lead to such symptoms as irascibility, insomnia and dreaminess, head distension, headache and dizziness.

1.1.2 Digestion

The liver's function of dredging and regulating can regulate qi activity and assist the spleen qi's elevating and stomach qi's descending, which is key to ensuring the normal digestive function of the spleen and stomach. In addition, it can promote the secretion of bile and the digestion of water and food. If the dredging and regulating function of the liver is abnormal, it often affects the digestive function of the spleen and stomach, bringing on the symptoms of belching, vomiting, nausea, abdominal pain and diarrhea, which is known as "liver qi attacking the stomach" and "disharmony between the liver and the spleen".

1.2 To store blood

The liver storing blood refers to the function of the liver to store blood and regulate the volume of blood. The blood in the human body often changes with different physiological activities. When the human body is moving, the blood tends to flow to the active tissues and organs, and the liver will output the stored blood to supply the body. During rest and sleep, a large amount of blood will flow into the liver.

1.3 To govern the tendons and the manifest externally on the nails

The tendons are the tissues that connect the joints and muscles. The liver governs the tendons, which means that the tendons of the whole body depends on the nourishment of liver blood. Only when liver blood is sufficient can the tendons get enough nourishment and function well. If the liver blood is deficient, the tendons cannot get enough nourishment, leading to numbness of the limbs, dysfunction of the joints, even tremor of hands and feet, convulsion of the limbs. The sufficiency or deficiency of liver blood can affect the color and quality of the nails.

1.4 To open into the eyes

"The liver opens into the eyes" means that the liver meridian runs upward into the eyes. The visual performance can be brought into full play only when the eyes are nourished by liver blood.

2. The heart

The heart is located in the chest and surrounded by the pericardium. Its main function is to govern blood and vessels and to control the mind.

2.1 To govern blood and vessels, manifesting on the face

The function of the heart to govern blood and vessels means that the heart propels blood to circulate in the vessels to nourish and moisten the body. The propelling of the blood circulating in the vessels depends on heart qi. If heart qi is vigrous, blood can circulate in the vessels continuously to meet the body's needs. Since the blood runs in the vessels and the blood vessels on the face are rich, the sufficiency or deficiency of heart qi will be reflected on the changes of pulse and complexion. If heart qi is vigorous and blood is sufficient, the pulse will be gentle and powerful and the complexion will be ruddy and lustrous; if heart qi is insufficient and the vessels are empty, the complexion will be pale and lusterless.

2.2 To control the mind

Mind refers to spirit, consciousness and thinking activities. According to modern physiology, spirit, consciousness and thinking activities are the functions of the brain, that is, the brain's response to the external objective things. In Chinese Medicine, it believes that mind is related to the five zang-organs and mainly belongs to the physiological function of the heart. If heart blood is insufficient, symptoms such as dysphoria, insomnia, dreaminess, amnesia and restlessness will often occur.

2.3 Opening into the tongue

The heart and the tongue are closely related in physiology. The heart meridian runs upward to the tongue, and heart qi and blood flow through the tongue. If the heart is diseased, it is often reflected on the tongue.

3. The spleen

The spleen is located in the middle energizer. Its main function is to transport and transform and to command blood.

3.1 The functions of transportation and transformation of the spleen include two aspects:

3.1.1 To transport and transform water and food essence

It mainly refers to the spleen's function of digesting, absorbing and transporting nutrients. Food enters the stomach and is digested by the stomach and spleen. The water and food essence in it are transported and distributed to the whole body through spleen qi to nourish the five zang-organs, six fu-organs, four limbs and bones, skin and hair, tendons and muscles. Since dietary water and food are the main source of nutrients needed by people after birth and the main material basis for the production of qi and blood, the spleen is called "the foundation of acquired constitution" and "the source of qi and blood". If spleen qi is healthy, the functions of digestion, absorption and distribution will be normal; if the spleen fails to transport and transform, it will lead to abdominal distension, loose stool, poor appetite, fatigue, emaciation, etc.

3.1.2 To transport and transform water

The spleen has the function of regulating the metabolism of water. Under the joint action the lung and kidney, it maintains the normal metabolism of the water in the body. If the spleen fails to function well, it may cause phlegm, edema and other symptoms of water retention.

3.2 To govern the muscles and four limbs

It means that the muscles and four limbs depend on the nutrients transported and transformed by the spleen to nourish. With normal function of the spleen and sufficient supply of nutrients, both the muscles and four limbs will become strong. If the function of the spleen is abnormal and the nourishment is insufficient, it will bring on the symptoms of emaciation or atrophy of the muscles and lassitude of the four limbs.

3.3 To command blood

To command means to control. To command blood means that the spleen controls blood circulation inside the vessels and prevents it from flowing out of the vessels. If spleen qi is weak and fails to command, blood will overflow the vessels, causing such symptoms as bloody stool, metrorrhagia, dermatorrhagia.

3.4 Opening into the mouth and manifesting on the lips

The idea that the spleen opens into the mouth means that the intake of food, appetite and taste in the mouth are closely related to the spleen's function of transportation and transformation. The changes of lips can reflect the state of spleen qi. If the spleen is normal in function, the appetite and taste in the mouth will be normal, and the lips will be ruddy, moist and lustrous. If the spleen is abnormal in function, it will lead to poor appetite, tastelessness in the mouth, lusterless and sallow lips. Therefore, the spleen "opens into the mouth and manifests on the lips".

4. The lung

The lung, including two lobes on the left and right, is located in the chest and above the heart. Its main function is to dominate qi and respiration, govern dispersion and descent, connect with all the vessels, and dominate regulation.

4.1 Dominating qi and respiration

The lung dominating qi includes two aspects.

4.1.1 To dominate respiration

The lung has the function of dominating respiration and is the place where air in and out of the body exchanges. The body inhales fresh air and exhales waste air through respiration of the lung to exchange air in and out of the body. In Yinyang Yingxiang Dalunpian (Major Discussion on the Theory of Yin and Yang and the Corresponding Relationships Among All the Things in Nature) of *Plain Questions*, "Tianqi (Heaven qi) communicates with the lung" is exactly what it means.

4.1.2 Dominating qi throughout the body

This is because the lung is closely related to the generation of pectoral qi. Pectoral qi is synthesized from the nutrients of food and fresh air inhaled by the lung, accumulating in the chest and distributing to the whole body through blood vessels to maintain the normal physiological activities of the body.

If the lung's function of regulating qi is normal, the airway is unobstructed and breathing is even. If lung qi is insufficient, it will not only weaken the respiratory function, but also affect the generation of pectoral qi, leading to symptoms due to qi deficiency such as weakness of breathing, shortness of breath and low voice.

4.2 To dominate dispersion and descent

Dispersion and descent of the lung are complementary. Harmonious dispersing and descending functions of the lung ensure even breathing, smooth water passage, normal circulation and distribution of water.

4.2.1 To dominate dispersion and associate with skin and hair externally

Dispersion means to diffuse and spread, that is, to distribute qi and body fluid upwards and outwards. The lung dominates dispersion, which means that the propelling of lung qi disperses defensive qi and body fluid to the whole body to warm and moisten the striae and interstitial space, skin and hair. The skin and hair are on the body surface, which is the barrier for the human body to resist invasion of external pathogens. Since the skin and hair are warmed and nourished by defensive qi and body fluid dispersed by the lung, the lung and skin and hair are closely related physiologically and pathologically. If lung qi is deficient and fails to disperse defensive qi and body fluid to the skin and hair, the skin and hair will become dry and malnourished, even susceptibility to external pathogens due to defensive qi's failure of consolidation.

4.2.2 To dominate descent and regulate water passage

Descent means the downward cleaning, that is, to disperse qi and body fluid downwards and inwards. The lung is located in the upper energizer. Lung qi functions to clean and descend. If lung qi fails to descend, it will lead to symptoms of chest oppression, cough and dyspnea due to upward flow of lung qi. At the same time, descent of lung qi ensures water from the upper energizer continuously infusing to the kidney and bladder and maintaining smooth urination.

4.3 Connecting with all the vessels and dominating regulation

"The lung is connected with all the vessels" means that through the vessels blood from the whole body passes the lung and after air exchanges through the lung's respiration, new blood is distributed to all parts of the body. "The lung dominates regulation" means that the lung has the function of regulating respiration and qi, blood, body fluid, water of the whole body. If lung qi is abundant, blood circulation and qi activity will be normal and smooth. If lung qi is deficient, heart blood will fail to flow and blood vessels will become stagnant, leading to symptoms such as palpitation, purplish tongue.

4.4 Opening into the nose

The ventilating and smelling functions of the nose mainly depend on the function of lung qi. If lung qi is harmonious, the respiration will be smooth and nose will be sensitive in smelling. If external pathogens invade the lung and lung qi fails to disperse, it will lead to symptoms such as nasal congestion, runny nose, insensitive smell; if lung heat is exuberant, it will lead to symptoms of dyspnea, flaring of nares. Therefore, the nose is regarded as the orifice into which the lung opens.

5. The kidney

The kidney is situated at either side of the spine in the lumbar region. Its main function is to store essence, govern water and receive qi.

5.1 To store essence

It means that the kidney governs growth and development, reproduction and qi activities of the viscera. The essence stored by the kidney includes congenital essence and acquired essence. The congenital essence inheriting from the parents is the basic material for growth, development and reproduction of the human body. Acquired essence comes from food nutrients transformed by the spleen and stomach, which is the basic substance for maintaining life activities of the human body. The congenital essence and acquired essence are interdependent and mutually promoting. The congenital essence must be supported by the acquired essence for continuous enrichment; the acquired essence must depend on the congenital essence for its production.

Essence can transform into qi, and qi transformed by kidney essence is called kidney qi. Kidney qi, produced by kidney essence and including kidney yin and kidney yang, can promote growth, development and reproduction of the human body. In childhood, kidney essence gradually becomes full; during adolescence, kidney qi enriches and sexual function gradually matures which indicates genitality; at the period of old age, the kidney essence gradually declines, the sexual function and genitality decline and disappear, and the body grows old. This process reflects the role of kidney essence in human growth, development and reproduction.For example, children's development retardation and certain infertility are manifestations of insufficient kidney essence.

5.2 To govern water

It means that the kidney controls and regulates the metabolism of water. The metabolism of water is related to the lung, spleen and kidney, and is mainly accomplished by the function of qi transformation of the kidney. Under normal circumstances, water is received by the stomach, transported by the spleen and distributed by the lung. The lucid part in water is transported by the triple energizer to various viscera; the turbid part is transformed into urine to be excreted out of the body. Thus relative equilibrium of water metabolism is maintained in the body. All these actions depend on the steaming action of kidney yang. If qi transformation of the kidney gets abnormal, it will bring on such disorders of water metabolism as difficult urination, edema.

5.3 To govern reception of qi

Although the respiratory function is controlled by the lung, the kidney has the function to receive lung qi. In other words, the kidney assists the lung to inhale qi which will be descended into the kidney. Only when kidney qi is sufficient and normal in receiving qi can the lung respire evenly and the air passage be clear. If kidney qi is deficient, it will bring on difficult respiration, frequent asthma, which is called "kidney fails to receive qi".

5.4 To govern bones, produce marrow, connect with the brain and manifest on the hair

The kidney stores essence and essence can produce marrow. Marrow is stored in the bones and nourishes the bones, so kidney essence is the material for the growth of bones. If kidney essence is sufficient, the production of bone marrow will be ensured and bones will be strong and powerful because of nourishment. If the kidney essence is deficient, the production of bone marrow will be reduced and symptoms of flaccidity of the skeleton, osteoporosis, maldevelopment will appear. Therefore, children with late closure of fontanel, flaccid and weak bones are mostly caused by insufficient kidney essence.

The marrow includes bone marrow and spinal cord. The spinal cord is connected with the brain which is the accumulation of marrow. That is why "brain is the sea of marrow". People's mental activities are mainly controlled by the heart, but they are also closely related to the brain. In Ming dynasty, Li Shizhen pointed out that : "The brain is the place where the primordial spirit is stored". Since the continuous production of brain marrow depends on kidney essence, people's mental activities are also related to the function of the kidney.

The hair depends on blood to nourish. That is why it is said that "the hair is the surplus of blood". However, hair needs to be nourished by kidney essence. Therefore, the growth and loss, nourishment and luster are associated with the state of kidney essence. Young adults have sufficient kidney essence, so their hair is black, thick and lustrous; the kidney qi of the elderly is weak, so their hair become white and easy to lose.

5.5 To open into the ears and dominate urination and defecation

The auditory function of the ears depend on the nourishment of kidney essence. If kidney qi is sufficient, hearing will be sensitive. If kidney essence is insufficient, symptoms such as tinnitus and hearing loss will occur. Deafness is common in the elderly because it is often due to deficiency of kidney essence.

Although the storage and excretion of urine is in the bladder, it depends on qi transformation of the kidney. If the kidney is deficient and qi transformation is abnormal, it will lead to difficult urination; if kidney deficiency fails to consolidate, it will bring on incontinence or enuresis. The evacuation of stools is also affected and controlled by kidney qi. Deficiency of kidney yang can cause constipation, and failure of consolidation by the kidney may cause prolonged ejaculation and spermatorrhea.

The Six Fu-organs

1. The gallbladder

The gallbladder is attached to the liver and stores bile which promotes the digestion and absorption of food. If the liver and gallbladder qi cannot disperse, dredge and descend or dampness-heat steams the liver and gallbladder, it will lead to bitter taste in the mouth, vomiting bitter water, or yellowish complexion and eyes due to upward flow of gallbladder qi and extravasation of bile. Although the gallbladder is one of the six fu-organs, it differs from other five organs but stores essence and does not receive water and food or waste. Therefore, it also belongs to extraordinary fu-organs.

2. The stomach

The stomach is located under the diaphragm, connected with the esophagus above and the small intestine below. The main physiological function of the stomach is to receive and decompose water and food. After being taken into the mouth, food passes through the esophagus and is received by the stomach, so the stomach is "the sea of food and water". The food in the stomach is decomposed into chyme and transmitted to the small intestine. Food essence is transported and transformed by the spleen to nourish the whole body, and this function is called "stomach qi action (digestive function)". The state of stomach qi affects both the gastrointestinal function and other viscera. In Chinese Medicine, it is attached much importance to the function of "stomach qi action" because the stomach is an important organ to receive, decompose and provide nutrition. That is why it is called "stomach qi action is the foundation of human body". In the observation of disease condition, it also emphasizes the functional state of the stomach. It is believed that "the existence of stomach qi action ensures life, while non-existence of stomach qi action leads to death", which is important to judge the prognosis of the disease.

3. The small intestine

The small intestine is connected with the stomach above and the large intestine below. Its main function is to separate the lucid from the turbid. The small intestine further digests the water and food transmitted from the stomach and separates the lucid from the turbid. The lucid is transported to the whole body by the spleen while the turbid is transmitted to the large intestine through the railing portal, and the surplus water infiltrates into the bladder. Therefore, the digestion and absorption of food and the excretion of urine and stools are closely related to the small intestine. If the small intestine is diseased, there will be abnormal urination and defecation in addition to its impact on the digestion and absorption function.

4. The large intestine

The large intestine is connected with the small intestine in the upper and the anus in the lower. Its main function is to transmit the waste. The large intestine receives the turbidity transmitted down from the small intestine, absorbs surplus water and transforms the food residues into feces to be discharged from the anus. If the large intestine is diseased, it will lead to abnormal transmission with such symptoms as constipation, dysentery, abdominal distension, diarrhea.

5. The bladder

The bladder is located in the lower abdomen. Its main function is to store and excrete urine. The bladder is one of the organs that dominate water metabolism. Water is distributed throughout the body through the actions of the spleen, lung, kidney and triple energizer. The metabolized water reaches the bladder through the water passage of triple energizer to become urine which is excreted out of the body through qi transformation of the bladder. If the qi transforming function of the bladder is abnormal, symptoms such as unsmooth urination, anuria may appear; if the bladder loses restraint, such symptoms as polyuria and urinary incontinence may appear.

6. The triple energizer

The triple energizer is a collective term of the upper, middle and lower energizer. Although the triple energizer belongs to one of the six fu-organs, it is not an independent organ but includes relevant viscera in the upper, middle and lower chest and abdomen and part of their functions. In terms of location, the part around stomach is the middle energizer, the part above it is the upper energizer and the part below it is the lower energizer. For the internal organs, the upper energizer includes the heart and the lung; the middle energizer includes the spleen and the stomach, and the lower energizer includes the liver, kidney, bladder.

Appendix: The uterus

The uterus is located in the lower abdomen and belongs to extraordinary fu-organs. It has the function of dominating menses and conceiving fetus.

The relationships among the zang-organs and the fu-organs

1. The relationships among the five zang-organs

1.1 The relationship between the heart and the lung

The heart dominates blood and the lung dominates qi. Coordination between the heart and the lung ensures normal circulation of qi and blood. If lung qi is too weak to propel heart blood, blood will not flow smoothly but become stagnant with symptoms of chest oppression, shortness of breath, palpitation, bluish lips and purplish tongue. If the function of the heart to govern blood declines and blood flow becomes unsmooth, it will affect the lung's dispersing and descending function, leading to symptoms of cough and asthma.

1.2 The relationship between the heart and the kidney

The heart is located in the upper and the kidney in the lower. The functions of them lie in the balance between heart yang and kidney water. If kidney water is insufficient and cannot nourish heart yin, symptoms such as palpitation, dysphoria and insomnia will occur; if heart yang is weak and heart fire cannot warm the kidney yang, it will lead to symptoms of palpitation and edema.

1.3 The relationship between the heart and the spleen

The heart governs blood and the spleen commands blood. If the function of the spleen is normal, the source of blood production will be sufficient and blood in the heart will be abundant. Blood runs in the vessels, which is propelled by heart qi and commanded by spleen qi. The coordination of the heart and the spleen ensures continuous production and normal circulation of blood. Dysfunction of the spleen will lead to insufficient source for blood production; failure of the spleen to command blood will lead to insufficient blood in the heart; overthinking will consume blood in the heart and affect the function of the spleen, leading to syndrome of deficiency of the heart and the spleen.

1.4 The relationship between the liver and the kidney

The liver stores blood and the kidney stores essence. Liver blood depends on the nourishment of kidney essence, and kidney essence also needs to be supplemented by the essence transformed by liver blood. Since essence and blood regenerate each other, there is a saying that "essence and blood are from the same source" and "the liver and the kidney are from the same source".

1.5 The relationship between the spleen and the kidney

The spleen is the acquired foundation of life while the kidney is the congenital foundation of life. The spleen's transporting and transforming function needs the assistance of the kidney yang's warming function; the innate essence of the kidney must rely on the supplement by the acquired water and food essence. The spleen and the kidney are mutually supplementing and promoting.

1.6 The relationship between the liver and the spleen

The liver governs dredging and dispersing and the spleen dominates transportation and transformation. They are closely related physiologically and mutually influential pathologically. The ascent and descent, transportation and transformation of the spleen and stomach depend on the dredging and dispersing of the liver qi. Only when the liver's dredging and dispersing function is normal can the spleen and stomach ascend and descend properly and transport and transform normally. If the relationship between them is unbalanced, symptoms such as chest and hypochondriac fullness, belching, vomiting, abdominal pain and diarrhea will occur.

2. The relationship between the five zang-organs and the six fu-organs

The relationship between the five zang-organs and the six fu-organs is mainly the "mutual internal and external relationship". The zang-organs pertain to yin while the fu-organs to yang. Yang manages the external while yin controls the internal. The internal and external relationship between the zang-organs and the fu-organs is realized by mutual association of the meridians. The exterior and interior are cooperative in physiology and mutually influential in pathology. They are introduced as follows:

2.1 The heart and the small intestine

The heart is related to the small intestine internally and externally. The relationship between the heart and the small intestine is quite obvious in pathology. If there is excess fire in the heart meridian, the heat can be shifted to the small intestine, leading to oliguria, brownish urine and burning sensation during urination; if there is heat in the small intestine, the heat can be shifted upward to the heart along the meridian, leading to dysphoria, reddish tongue and sores in the mouth.

2.2 The lung and the large intestine

The lung and the large intestine are related internally and externally. Normal function of the lung to purify and descend promotes the normal transmitting function of the large intestine. the transmitting function of the large intestine will be normal; smooth transmission of the large intestine also promotes purification and descent of lung qi. If the lung fails to purify and descend, it will affect the transmission of the large intestine, leading to difficult defecation and abdominal distension; if the large intestine is obstructed, it will lead to failure of lung qi to descend, leading to cough, asthma, chest fullness, etc.

2.3 The spleen and the stomach

The spleen and the stomach are related internally and externally. The spleen governs transportation and transformation while the stomach controls reception. Ascent ensures normal function of the spleen and descent harmonizes the function of the stomach. Ascent of spleen qi ensures elevation of water and food essence; descent of stomach qi ensures downward transmission of water and food. The spleen pertains to yin, preferring dryness and disliking dampness; the stomach pertains to yang, preferring moisture and disliking dryness. The spleen and the stomach are related by coordination between yin and yang, mutually influencing by ascent and descent, mutually promoting between dryness and dampness, and thus they complete the digestion and absorption of food as well as the transportation and distribution of water and food essence.

2.4 The liver and the gallbladder

The gallbladder attaches to the liver with which it is internally and externally related. Normal dispersing and dredging function of the liver ensures smooth excretion of bile; normal excretion of bile promotes the liver's dispersing and dredging function. Therefore, they are closely related. The liver and the gallbladder also affect each other pathologically, leading to simultaneous disorder of them such as exuberant fire of the liver and the gallbladder, dampness-heat of the liver and the gallbladder.

2.5 The kidney and the bladder

The kidney and the bladder are related internally and externally. The qi transforming function of the bladder is closely related to kidney qi. If kidney qi is sufficient, qi transforming function of the bladder will be normal and the bladder will open and close properly to ensure normal function of storing and excreting urine; if kidney qi is insufficient, qi transforming function will be abnormal and the bladder will not open and close properly, leading to dysuria or incontinence, enuresis and frequent urination. Therefore, disorders related to the storage and excretion of urine are mostly related to the kidney in addition to the bladder itself.

3. The relationships among the six fu-organs

The main function of the six fu-organs is to transmit and transform. The six fu-organs coordinate in the whole process of food digestion, absorption and excretion. Food enters the stomach and then is decomposed and transmitted downward to the small intestine. The gallbladder excretes bile which enters the small intestine to promote digestion. After primary digestion in the stomach, food is transmitted to the small intestine where the chyme is further digested by separating the lucid from the turbid. The lucid nourishes the whole body while the turbid enters the large intestine and water infiltrates into the bladder; the waste in the large intestine is further absorbed and the residues (feces) will be excreted out of the body; water infiltrates into the bladder and becomes urine which is excreted out of the body by qi transforming action. The whole process of digestion, absorption and excretion depends on the qi transforming and water-passage-dredging function of the triple energizer.

It can been seen that there are close relationships among the six fu-organs in physiology. The six fu-organs also affect each other pathologically. If one fu-organ is diseased, it will affect other fu-organs. For instance, if excess heat in the stomach consumes body fluid, it will lead to dry stools and unsmooth transmission of the large intestine; dryness of the large intestine and absence of defecation will also affect the descent of stomach qi, leading to upward flow of stomach qi with symptoms of nausea and vomiting.

Section 2 Meridians, Collaterals and Meridian System

The meridians and collaterals

The meridians and collaterals are important components of the body. They distribute all over the body, connecting the internal viscera with the external tissues and organs into an organic whole. They are the pathways through which the human body transports qi and blood.

The theory of the meridians is an important part of the basic theory of traditional Chinese medicine (Chinese Medicine). For a long time, it has been guiding the clinical practice of various departments of Chinese medicine; it is especially significant in acupuncture, moxibustion and Tuina. In recent years, many new therapies have been developed based on the theory of the meridians, such as acupuncture anesthesia, water acupuncture therapy, catgut embedding therapy and acupoint ligation therapy, which also enrich the theory of the meridians.

1.The concept of meridians and collaterals

It is a collective term for the meridians and collaterals. The meridian means route. The meridians are the main straight trunks, such as the twelve regular meridians. Collateral means "network". The collaterals are the branches of the meridians, including divergent collaterals, superficial collaterals and fine collaterals. They are criss-crossed and connect the whole body into a network.

The meridians and collaterals are the pathways for qi and blood to circulate in the whole body. These pathways connect the interior with the exterior, link the upper part with the lower part of the body, and associate the internal with the external, thus regulating various parts in the body. The meridians and collaterals connect the tissues and organs of the five zang-organs, six fu-organs, four limbs and skeletons, five sensory organs and nine orifices into an organic whole.

2. The composition of the meridian system

It is composed of the meridians and the collaterals. The meridians can be classified into two categories, namely the twelve regular meridians and the eight extraordinary meridians, which are the main parts of the meridian system. The twelve regular meridians include three yin meridians of Taiyin, Shaoyin and Jueyin of the hand and foot respectively, and three yang meridians of Taiyang, Shaoyang and Yangming of the hand and foot respectively. The eight extraordinary meridians include governor vessel, conception vessel, thoroughfare vessel, belt vessel, yin heel vessel, yang heel vessel, yin link vessel and yang link vessel. The collaterals are divided into divergent collaterals, superficial collaterals and fine collaterals. The divergent collaterals are large. Each of the twelve regular meridians has one divergent collateral and so do the governor vessel and conception vessel. Together with the large spleen collateral, there are "fifteen divergent collaterals". The floating collaterals running in the shallow regions of the body are called "superficial collaterals". The smallest branches of the collaterals are called "fine collaterals".

In addition, there are twelve branches of the meridians, the twelve meridian sinews and the twelve skin divisions.

3. The functions of the meridians and collaterals

3.1 Physiological aspect

The meridians and collaterals have the function to connect the exterior with the interior, associate the viscera with other organs, transport qi and blood, defend the exogenous pathogens and protect the body. The tissues and organs of the five zang-organs, six fu-organs, four limbs, nine orifices, skin, muscle, tendons and bones have different physiological functions, but they make the body coordinated as an organic whole. The mutual connection and organic cooperation are mainly realized by the communication function of the meridian system. At the same time, the meridians are the pathways for qi and blood circulation. With propelling of heart qi, qi and blood flow all around the body to nourish various tissues and organs, and play a role in resisting exogenous pathogens and protecting the body, thus maintaining normal physiological activities of the body.

3.2 Pathological aspect

Pathologically, the meridians and collaterals are mainly related to the occurrence and transmission of disease. When healthy qi is insufficient and the meridians lose their normal functions, the body will be susceptible to the exogenous pathogenic factors and thus disease occurs. After a disease occurs, pathogens are often transmitted from the external to the internal, from the exterior to the interior along the meridians and collaterals. Therefore, physiologically the meridians and collaterals are pathways for the circulation of qi and blood, and pathologically they are also pathways for the development and transformation of diseases.

The meridians and collaterals are not only the pathways for the transmission of exogenous pathogens from the exterior into the interior, but also important channels for the mutual influence of the pathological changes among the viscera and between the viscera and the external tissues and organs. The visceral disorders can affect each other through the connection of meridians and collaterals. For instance, liver disease affects the stomach, heart disease transfers heat to the small intestine, etc. The visceral disorders can be reflected on certain parts of the body surface, such as red, swelling and painful eyes due to liver fire, deafness due to gallbladder fire, and earache.

3.3 Diagnostic aspect

The meridians pertain to the viscera, and there are fixed running routes on the body surface. Therefore, visceral diseases can be reflected on relevant meridians. Clinically, the diagnosis of a disease is often based on the symptoms of the disease, combination with the running routes of the meridians and collaterals, and their pertaining relationship to certain viscera. For example, hypochondriac pain indicates liver and gallbladder disease; lumbago is usually related to kidney disease. Diseases of different viscera show special reaction points on certain acupoints which pertain to corresponding viscera. For example, lung disease will bring on tenderness on Zhongfu (LU 1); appendicitis will cause tenderness on Lanwei (EX-LE7). Besides, the diagnosis of certain diseases can also be based on the running route and distribution laws of the meridians. Take headache for example. Pain of the forehead is related to Yangming meridian; pain on both sides of the head is usually related to Shaoyang meridian; pain on the nape is related to Taiyang meridian; pain on the top of the head is related to Jueyin meridian.

3.4 Treatment

The theory of the meridians is widely applied to clinical treatments, and it has great guiding significance for acupuncture and moxibustion, massage and drug therapy.

In terms of drug therapy, since some drugs have special therapeutic effects on certain viscera, meridians and collaterals, Chinese Medicine has developed the theory of "meridian tropism of drugs", which plays a guiding role in the clinical application of drugs. For example, all the three drugs of Qianghuo (Rhizoma et Radix Notopterygii), Baizhi (Radix Angelicae Dahuricae) and Chaihu (Radix Bupleuri) can treat headache. Howerver, Qianghuo (Rhizoma et Radix Notopterygii) is used for Taiyang headache; Baizhi (Radix Angelicae Dahuricae) is used for Yangming headache and Chaihu (Radix Bupleuri) is used for Shaoyang headache. For another example, the three drugs of Huanglian (Rhizoma Coptidis), Huangqin (Radix Scutellariae) and Huangbai (Cortex Phellodendri Chinensis) can clear away heat. However, Huanglian (Rhizoma Coptidis) is effective for clearing away heat in the heart; Huangqin (Radix Scutellariae) is effective for clearing away heat in the lung and Huangbai (Cortex Phellodendri Chinensis) is effective for clearing away heat in the kidney.

In acupuncture treatment, the method of "selection of acupoints along the meridians" is often applied to treat disease of a certain organ or tissue. For example, Zusanli (ST 36) is often selected for stomachache; Qimen (LR 14) of the liver meridian is often selected for liver disease. At present, acupuncture anesthesia, widely applied in surgery, is also developed on the basis of the theory of the meridians. It achieves anesthesia and analgesia by needling certain meridian acupoints.

Other therapies such as Tuina and Qigong also widely apply the theory of the meridians.

The twelve meridians

1. The naming of the twelve meridians

The naming of the twelve meridians is based on the name of the viscera, the running regions and the theory of yin and yang. For example, the meridian associated with the heart is called the "heart meridian", and the meridian associated with the lung is called the "lung meridian". The meridian running mainly in the upper limbs is called the "hand meridian" while the meridian running mainly in the lower limbs is called the "foot meridian". The one associated with the zang-organ is "yin meridian" while the one associated with the fu-organ is "yang meridian". For example, lung meridian of hand Taiyin means that this meridian runs in the upper limbs, pertaining to the lung which belongs to five zang-organs and pertains to yin.

Classification Table of the Names of the Twelve Meridians

Hand and foot attribution and circulation	Yin meridians (pertaining to zang-organs)	Yang meridians (pertaining to fu-organs)	Main circulation parts: Yin meridians run on the medial side while yang meridians run on the lateral side	
Hand	Lung meridian of Taiyin	Large intestine meridian of Yangming	Upper limbs	Anterior line
	Pericardium meridian of Jueyin	Triple energizer meridian of Shaoyang		Midline
	Heart meridian of Shaoyin	Small intestine meridian of Taiyang		Posterior line
Foot	Spleen meridian of Taiyin	Stomach meridian of Yangming	Lower limbs	Anterior line
	Liver meridian of Jueyin	Gallbladder meridian of Shaoyang		Midline
	Kidney meridian of Shaoyin	Bladder meridian of Taiyang		Posterior line

Note: In the lower part of the lower leg and the dorsum of the foot, the liver meridian is on the anterior line and the spleen meridian is on the midline. The two meridians cross about 8 cun above tip of internal malleolus, and then the spleen meridian runs to the anterior and the liver meridian runs to the midline.

2. The running direction, crossing, distribution law and flowing order of the twelve meridians

2.1 The running direction, crossing and distribution law

The twelve meridians include three yin meridians of the hand, three yang meridians of the hand, three yang meridians of the foot and three yin meridians of the foot. The running direction, crossing and distribution laws: The three yin meridians of the hand run from the chest to the hand and converge with the three yang meridians of the hand; the three yang meridians of the hand run from the hand to the head and converge with the three yang meridians of the foot; the three yang meridians of the foot run from the head to the foot and converge with the three yin meridians of the foot; the three yin meridians of the foot run from the foot to the abdomen and converge with the three yin meridians of the hand.

From the above laws, it can be seen that the yang meridians converge over the head and face; the yin meridians converge over the chest and abdomen; the yin meridians and yang meridians converge over the end of the four limbs.

The yin meridians distribute along the interior of the four limbs. The order: Taiyin meridian distributes along the anterior border, Jueyin meridian along the midline and Shaoyin meridian along the posterior border. Over the interior side of the lower leg, Jueyin meridian and Taiyin meridian cross about 8 cun above the tip of internal malleolus. Taiyin meridian distributes along the anterior border, Jueyin meridian along the midline and Shaoyin along the posterior border. The yang meridians distribute on the lateral side of the four limbs. The order: Yangming meridian distributes along the anterior border, Shaoyang meridian along the midline and Taiyang meridian along the posterior border.

2.2 The external and internal relationships and circulation order

The twelve meridians are related to the six zang-organs (including pericardium) and six fu-organs, constituting six pairs of meridians which are internally and externally related. The lung meridian of hand Taiyin and the large intestine meridian of hand Yangming are related internally and externally; the heart meridian of hand Shaoyin and the small intestine meridian of hand Taiyang are related internally and externally; the pericardium meridian of hand Jueyin and the triple energizer meridian of hand Shaoyang are related internally and externally; the spleen meridian of foot Taiyin and the stomach meridian of foot Yangming are related internally and externally; the kidney meridian of foot Shaoyin and the bladder meridian of foot Taiyang are related internally and externally; the liver meridian of foot Jueyin and the gallbladder meridian of foot Shaoyang are related internally and externally. The external and internal relationship manifests on two aspects: For one thing, the viscera are interrelated internally and externally. Yin meridians pertain to the zang-organs and connect the fu-organs with their collaterals while yang meridians pertain to the fu-organs and connect the zang-organs with their collaterals. For another, the meridians in external and internal relationship are connected with each other at the extremities of the four limbs. Yin meridians of the hand connect with yang meridians while yang meridians of the foot connect with yin meridians. Since there are internal and external relationships among the twelve meridians of the hands and feet, they are interrelated physiologically and mutually influential pathologically.

The twelve meridians are distributed in the interior and exterior of the body. Qi and blood flow in the meridians following a circular and infusing order: Starting from the lung meridian of hand Taiyin, transmitting to the liver meridian of foot Jueyin and then the lung meridian of hand Taiyin. This cycle is endless. The flowing and infusing order of the twelve meridians is demonstrated in the following: The lung meridian of hand Taiyin→the large intestine meridian of hand Yangming→the stomach meridian of foot Yangming→the spleen meridian of foot Taiyin→the heart meridian of hand Shaoyin→the small intestine meridian of hand Taiyang→the bladder meridian of foot Taiyang→the kidney meridian of foot Shaoyin→the pericardium meridian of hand Jueyin→the triple energizer meridian of hand Shaoyang→the gallbladder meridian of foot Shaoyang→the liver meridian of foot Jueyin→the lung meridian of hand Taiyin.

The eight extraordinary vessels

The eight extraordinary vessels include governor vessel, conception vessel, thoroughfare vessel, belt vessel, yin heel vessel, yang heel vessel, yin link vessel and yang link vessel. Compared with the twelve regular meridians, they have no direct connection with the viscera or internal and external relationship between each other, so they are called "extraordinary vessels". The eight extraordinary vessels run around among the twelve meridians with the functions of strengthening the connection among the meridians and regulating qi and blood of the twelve meridians. The four vessels of governor vessel, conception vessel, thoroughfare vessel and belt vessel which have close relationship with the clinical practice will be introduced as follows:

1. The governor vessel

The governor vessel governs all yang meridians in the body. The three yang meridians of the hands and feet in the twelve meridians all converge at the governor vessel, so the governor vessel is known as "the sea of yang meridians".

2. The conception vessel

The conception vessel has the function of governing all yin meridians of the body, so it is known as "the sea of yin meridians". The conception vessel starts from the uterus and has the function of conceiving fetus, so it is known as "the conception vessel dominating uterus and gestation".

3. The thoroughfare vessel

The thoroughfare vessel has the function of controlling qi and blood of the whole body and is the major route for qi and blood circulation, so it is known as "the sea of the twelve meridians" and "the sea of blood".

4. The belt vessel

The belt vessel starts from the hypochondria and runs transversely around the waist and abdomen like a belt. That is why it is called belt vessel. The belt vessel has the function to control yin and yang meridians, so there is a saying that "all the meridians and vessels are controlled by the belt vessel". Disharmony of the belt vessel often leads to various gynecological diseases.

The unique application of Back-Shu acupoints

The bladder meridian of foot Taiyang starts from Jingming (BL 1) of the inner canthus, ascends to the forehead and joins the governor vessel at the vertex. From there it enters the brain, reemerges and runs downwards and along the medial side of the scapular region. Then it runs along the spinal column, which is one of the major meridians on the back, including 18 pairs of Shu acupoints. Back-Shu acupoints are special acupoints where qi of the viscera is infused. The distribution order of Back-Shu acupoints is similar to that of the locations of the zang-organs and fu-organs. They can reflect the visceral disorders and can be used to treat visceral disorders.

Five Zang-Organ Shu acupoints and Geshu (BL17)

The so-called Shu acupoints refer to the acupoints on the back where visceral qi is infused. In other words, the meridian qi of the viscera is infused here, and the state of visceral qi and blood can be manifested on corresponding Shu acupoints.

The gallbladder meridian of foot Taiyang is in the exterior and pertains to yang while five zang-organs are in the interior and pertains to yin. According to Yinyang Yingxiang Dalunpian (Major Discussion on the Theory of Yin and Yang and the Corresponding Relationships Among All the Things in Nature) of *Plain Questions*: "Those who are good at acupuncture are often trying to draw yang from yin, draw yin from yang, needle the acupoints located on the right side to treat diseases on the left side and needle the acupoints located on the left side to treat diseases on the right side. By comparing the normal conditions of themselves with the abnormal conditions of the patients, they understand the pathological changes of the patients; by examining the manifestations in the exterior they know the pathological changes in the interior. These are the methods they use to judge excess and deficiency. From small signs they can decide the location of diseases. This attitude toward treatment will prevent diseases from turning fatal". For the meaning of "drawing yang from yin, drawing yin from yang", Zhang Zhicong explained that: "All of these yin and yang, qi and blood, exterior and interior, left and right are mutually permeated, so those who are good at acupuncture are often trying to draw pathogen of yang phase from yin and draw pathogen of yin phase from yang."

Among the Five Zang-Organ Shu acupoints, Feishu (BL 13) is of the highest position and located below and 1.5 cun lateral to the third thoracic vertebra. The lung governs qi throughout the body, respiration, skin and hair, the opening and closing of the striae and interstices. The lung and defensive qi are the first to be attacked when the exogenous pathogenic factors attack. Lung qi deficiency leads to emptiness of Feishu (BL 13). Needling Feishu (BL 13) can disperse lung qi, clear away heat and harmonize nutrient phase, supplement lung qi and regulate qi. Xinshu (BL 15) is located below and 1.5 cun lateral to the spinous process of the fifth thoracic vertebra. The heart dominates blood and stores spirit. Insufficiency of heart qi and heart blood will lead to emptiness of Xinshu (BL 15). Needling Xinshu (BL 15) has the function of regulating blood and harmonizing nutrient phase and tranquilizing the mind. Ganshu (BL 18) is located below and 1.5 cun lateral to the spinous process of the ninth thoracic vertebra. Liver stores blood and functions to dredge and regulate. The liver prefers to grow freely and dominates tendons. Transverse flow of liver qi attacks the stomach and the liver fails to store blood, which will lead to blood extravasation and nasal bleeding. Liver blood deficiency leads to emptiness of Ganshu (BL 18). Needling of Ganshu (BL 18) has the function of soothing the liver and relieving depression, harmonizing blood and calming the mind. Pishu (BL 20) is located below and 1.5 cun lateral to the spinous process of the eleventh thoracic vertebra. The spleen governs transportation and transformation and controls blood. Failure of transportation due to spleen deficiency may lead to dysfunction. The spleen and the stomach are related internally and externally. Coordination of the upper and the lower leads to smooth qi movement. Obstruction of the middle energizer leads to dysfunction of ascending and descending. Spleen qi deficiency leads to empty Pishu (BL 20). Needling Pishu (BL 20) has the functions of strengthening the spleen and removing dampness, harmonizing the stomach and regulating the middle energizer, coordinating the ascending and descending function. Shenshu (BL 23) is located below and 1.5 cun lateral to the spinous process of the second lumbar vertebra. The kidney stores essence and dominates fire of life gate, and it is the residence of primordial yin and primordial yang. According to

Jing Yue Quan Shu (*Jingyue's Complete Works*): "Life gate is the sea of essence and blood, and the spleen and stomach are the sea of water and food; both of them are the roots of the five zang-organs and six fu-organs. However, life gate is the root of primordial qi and residence of water of fire. Yin qi of the five zang-organs relies on it to be nourished; yang qi of the five zang-organs relies on it to disperse; the spleen and stomach as the earth of middle energizer cannot produce without fire." Deficiency of the kidney means failure of the five-zang organs to store essence. Decline of fire of life gate will lead to failure of the five zang-organs and six fu-organs to disperse yang qi and emptiness of Shenshu (BL 23). Needling Shenshu (BL 23) has the function of supplementing kidney qi and essence and benefiting yin. The mutual generation and restriction and functional coordination among the five zang-organs ensures full vitality. Disharmony among the five zang-organs leads to various diseases.

Geshu (BL 17) is among the 18 pairs of Shu acupoints of the bladder meridian of the foot Taiyang, which is one of the eight confluent acupoints. "Blood converges at Geshu (BL 17)." Needling Geshu (BL 17) has the functions of regulating blood and qi, ascending the lucid and descending the turbid, and promoting flow of qi and blood, which has the general function of treating all blood diseases. Therefore, the overall functions of the Five Zang-Organ Shu acupoints plus Geshu (BL 17) include consolidating the five zang-organs, regulating qi and harmonizing blood, supplementing healthy qi and regulating yin and yang.

Section 3 Routine Operations of Chinese Medicine Diagnosis

Diagnosis is a method of examining diseases, including inspection, auscultation and olfaction, inquiry, pulse-taking and palpation, also known as four diagnostic methods.

When performing diagnosis, the doctor should be careful and meticulous. "To synthesize the four diagnostic methods" is to determine the cause, nature and internal relationship by understanding the external symptoms and signs from the perspective of the concept of holism, and thus to ensure comprehensive analysis and correct judgment and provide reliable basis for syndrome differentiation and treatment.

Inspection

Inspection refers to purposeful observation of the patient's spirit, complexion, shape, posture, tongue, etc. to understand the condition of the disease, including the inspection of the whole body and the local regions. In medical practice, people have gradually realized that certain changes of qi, blood, yin and yang in the viscera can be reflected on the outside of the human body, especially on the face and tongue. Therefore, some diseases inside the body can be understood through inspection.

1. Inspection of the whole body

1.1 Inspection of the spirit

Spirit refers to general manifestation of life activities, including spirit, consciousness and thinking. The material basis of spirit is essence. Inspection of the spirit mainly focuses on the examination of the mental state and conscious activity, speech and breath to determine the state of qi, blood, yin and yang of the viscera, severity and the prognosis of the disease.

Generally speaking, exuberant essence ensures full vitality while declined essence leads to poor vitality. Existence of spirit manifests as flexible eyes with brightness and vitality, clear mind and speech, sensitive response, which suggests non-impairment of healthy qi, mild pathological condition and favourable prognosis. Loss of spirit, also known as depletion of spirit, manifests as dull eye expression, low voice, retarded response or even unconsciousness or coma, and carphology, which indicates impairment of healthy qi, serious disease with unfavourable prognosis.

1.2 Inspection of the complexion

It means to observe the color and luster of the face. The color and luster of the face is the external reflection of visceral qi and blood. Therefore, the changes of the disease condition can be inferred through the inspection of the complexion.

1.3 Inspection of the body

It means to observe the physical obesity, emaciation, weakness and strength of the patient to understand the states of the constitution and conditions of the visceral qi and blood. Those with strong physique, thick bones, wide chest, strong muscles, moist and lustrous skin indicate exuberant qi and blood; those with thin body, bones and chest, lean muscles, dry and lusterless skin indicate deficiency of qi and blood.

1.4 Inspection of the postures

It means to examine the patient's postures in tranquility and action as well as the changes of body position related to the disease to know the internal disease. Different diseases may be reflected by different postures and positions. Preference for movement and speech indicates disease of yang nature while preference for tranquility indicates disease of yin nature. Lying on bed facing the outward with the ability to turn the body freely usually indicates yang syndrome, heat syndrome and excess syndrome; lying on bed facing the inward with inability to turn the body freely indicates yin syndrome, cold syndrome and deficiency syndrome; lying on a supine position with the extension of the limbs and refusal to cover quilt or put on clothes indicates heat syndrome; huddling up when lying on bed with preference to put on more clothes and warm by a fire indicates cold syndrome.

2. Inspection of the local regions

2.1 Inspection of the head and hair

It means to understand the conditions of the kidney, qi and blood by observing the head and hair of the patient.

Bigger head or smaller head with low intelligence in children is usually caused by insufficiency of kidney essence; sunken fontanel indicates deficiency syndrome; protrusion of fontanel indicates heat syndrome; retarded closure of the fontanel with weak neck indicates kidney qi deficiency.

Sparse hair is easy to lose or dry and lusterless hair often indicates essence and blood deficiency; sudden patch loss of hair is often caused by blood deficiency and wind attack.

2.2 Inspection of the eyes

The eyes are the orifices related to the liver. However, all visceral essence flows upward into the eyes. Therefore, diseases of the eyes are not only related to the liver but also reflect the disorder of other viscera. Redness and swelling of the eyes often indicates wind heat or liver fire; yellowish white part indicates jaundice; pale canthus indicates qi and blood deficiency; red and ulcerated canthus often indicates dampness-heat; puffiness of the eyelid indicates edema; sunken orbit is often due to loss of body fluid.

2.3 Inspection of the mouth and lips

It means to observe the changes of the color, dryness, moisture and shape. For example, pale mouth and lips often indicate blood deficiency; bluish and purplish lips indicate cold coagulation and blood stasis; dark red and dry lips indicate exuberant heat impairing body fluid; bright red lips indicate yin deficiency and hyperactive fire; ulcerated mouth and lips indicate heat accumulation in the spleen and stomach; distortion of the corners of the mouth indicates stroke.

2.4 Inspection of the teeth

Teeth are the surplus of bones and gums are connected with the collaterals of the stomach. Attention should be paid to the color and local changes. Dry teeth often indicate exuberant stomach fire; loose and sparse teeth and exposure of the root of tooth often indicate kidney deficiency or up-flaming of deficient fire; gritting teeth during sleep usually indicates indigestion or parasitic malnutrition; white gums often indicate up-flaming of stomach fire.

2.5 Inspection of the throat

Attention should be paid to the abnormal changes of the color and shape. Reddish, swollen and painful throat is due to stagnant heat in the lung and stomach; reddish swelling and ulceration of the throat with yellowish white suppurative points indicates extreme exuberance of heat virulence in the lung and stomach; bright red and tender throat with slight pain is due to yin deficiency and hyperactive fire; false whitish membrane which is not erasable on the throat, bleeding when rubbed heavily and reappearing is diphtheria.

2.6 Inspection of the macules and eruptions

Attention should be paid to the changes of color and shape. Macules refer to reddish even patches underneath the skin that cannot fade when pressed. Eruptions refer to reddish points like millet that can be felt by hands and fade when pressed.

3. Inspection of the tongue

Inspection of the tongue is an important part of inspection diagnosis in Chinese Medicine. The visceral disorders can be reflected by the tongue states.

Inspection of the tongue mainly includes observation of the tongue body and inspection of the tongue coating. The body of the tongue is composed of muscles and vessels. Tongue coating, produced by stomach qi, is a layer of fur attached to the surface of the tongue. Normal states of the tongue: the normal states of the tongue are marked by softness, flexibility, light-red color, even and whitish thin tongue coating which is neither too dry nor too moist and attached to the surface of the tongue. It is generally called "light-reddish tongue with thin and whitish fur".

Since certain parts of the tongue are related to the viscera and reflect the pathological changes of relevant viscera, the tongue is divided into the tip of the tongue, the center of the tongue, the root of the tongue, the margins of the tongue, which corresponds to the heart and lung, the spleen and stomach, the kidney, the liver and gallbladder respectively.

Methods and precautions for the inspection of the tongue: Tongue diagnosis should be performed in sufficient natural light. The patient should open the mouth and protrude the tongue naturally. Inspect of the tongue coating first, then the tip, center, root and margins of the tongue. Then observe the tongue body from the tip to the margins of the tongue. The inspection should be quick. If necessary, repeat the inspection once to twice.

In addition, pay attention to "dyed tongue coating" or other false manifestations. For example, ebony, olive, etc. can blacken the tongue coating; Chinese medicine such Huanglian (Rizoma Coptidis), Huangbai (Cortex Phellodendri Chinensis) can make the tongue coating yellow; overheated diet can make the tongue red; scraping the tongue can make the tongue coating from thick to thin. Therefore, in the inspection of the tongue, in addition to paying attention to the method of tongue extension and light, it is also necessary to pay attention to the influence of other factors in order to obtain correct observation results.

3.1 Inspection of the tongue quality

It means to inspect the changes of the color and the shape of the tongue, which indicates the diseases of visceral qi and blood.

3.1.1 Inspection of the color of the tongue

The tongue lighter than normal in color is called pale tongue. It indicates cold syndrome and deficiency syndrome which is often caused by declined yang qi and insufficient qi and blood.

The tongue darker than normal in color is called red tongue which usually indicates heat syndrome.

The deep or dull red tongue is called deep-red tongue which often indicates exuberant heat.

Purplish tongue often indicates blood stasis.

3.1.2 Inspection of the shape of the tongue

The tongue bigger than usual is called bulgy tongue. Pale and bulgy tongue is often due to yang deficiency of the spleen and the kidney; dark red and bulgy tongue is often caused by exuberant heat of the heart and the spleen.

The tongue thinner than usual is called thin and emaciated tongue, indicating deficiency of yin blood. Light-colored and thin tongue is often caused by deficiency of the heart and spleen, deficiency of qi and blood; deep-red and thin tongue is caused by exuberant heat consuming yin, and this condition is relatively serious.

Tongue with various fissures is called fissured tongue. Deep-red and fissured tongue is due to exuberant heat consuming fluid; light-colored and fissured tongue is due to deficiency of qi and blood.

Tooth-marked tongue means that the margins of the tongue are printed with tooth marks. The bulgy tongue squeezed by teeth causes tooth-marked tongue. Tooth-marked tongue and bulgy tongue appear simultaneously, indicating spleen deficiency and excessive dampness.

Prickly tongue refers to the tongue with hyperplasia and bulgy lingual papillae which look like pricks, indicating internal accumulation of pathogenic heat.

3.2 Inspection of the tongue coating includes examination of the changes of the nature and color of the tongue coating

3.2.1 Inspection of the color of the tongue coating

White tongue coating indicates exterior syndrome and cold syndrome.

Yellow tongue coating indicates heat syndrome and interior syndrome. The yellower the tongue coating, the greater the pathogenic heat.

Grayish tongue coating indicates interior syndrome, which can be seen in interior-heat syndrome or cold-dampness syndrome.

Black tongue coating indicates interior syndrome, extreme heat, or excessive cold, which is commonly seen in the severe stage of a disease.

3.2.2 Inspection of the nature of the tongue coating

Moistening and dryness of the tongue coating. The moistening and dryness of the tongue coating reflects the changes of body fluid. Tongue coating with too much water is called slippery tongue coating, indicating internal exuberance of water dampness; the tongue coating that is dry is called dry tongue coating, often indicating exuberant heat impairing body fluid or insufficiency of yin fluid.

Greasy and putrid tongue coating. Loose, sparse, thick tongue coating which is like soybean curb residues and easy to exfoliate is called putrid tongue coating; slippery and sticky tongue coating which is difficult to exfoliate is called greasy tongue coating, often seen in syndromes due to dampness, phlegm and fluid retention, food retention.

Auscultation and Olfaction

Auscultation and olfaction means listening to the sounds and smelling the odor to infer the pathological condition. Listening to the sounds is mainly to listen to the changes of patient's speech, breath and cough. Smelling the odor is mainly to smell the abnormal odor from the mouth, secreta and excreta.

1. Listening to the sounds

1.1 Listening to the voice

The strength of the patient's voice reflects the state of healthy qi and is also related to the nature of pathogenic qi. For example, sonorous voice with restlessness and polylogia indicates excess syndrome and heat syndrome; low and weak voice with quietness and oligologia indicates deficiency syndrome and cold syndrome.

1.2 Listening to the respiration

Weak breath and shortness of breath with low voice are often due to internal injury and consumption; powerful rapid breath with high voice is usually due to exuberant endogenous heat. Dyspnea refers to difficulty in breath, opening the mouth and raising the shoulders, inability to lie flat. Dyspnea is either of deficiency or excess nature. Excess dyspnea is marked by rapid and deep breath; deficient dyspnea is marked by slow and weak breath, less inhalation and more exhalation, and discontinued breath.

1.3 Listening to the cough

Deep cough often pertains to excess syndrome while cough with low voice and weak breath usually pertains to deficiency syndrome; cough with yellowish thick sputum difficult to expectorate is often due to lung heat; cough with profuse whitish sputum easy to expectorate is usually due to stagnation of cold phlegm or damp phlegm in the lung; dry cough without sputum or with scanty sticky phlegm is often due to dryness attacking the lung or yin deficiency and lung dryness.

2. Olfaction

Foul breath is usually due to stomach heat or indigestion, or dental caries, unclean mouth; sour odor from the mouth indicates retention of food in the stomach; stinking and foul sputum with pus and blood is usually seen in lung abscess; discharge of foul and thick snivel suggests nasosinusitis due to lung heat; stinking and turbid urine indicates downward migration of dampness-heat; sour and foul flatus indicates retention of food; foul menorrhea indicates heat and stinking menorrhea indicates cold; foul and thick leukorrhea is often due to dampness-heat; stinking leukorrhea usually pertains to deficient cold syndrome.

Inquiry

Inquiry is a diagnostic method to purposefully inquire the patient or his or her companion by the doctor. Patient's general condition, history of present illness, anamnesis, personal history and family history should be understood through inquiry.

The purpose of inquiry is to collect data related to syndrome differentiation and treatment to understand the location, nature, etiology as well as the states of healthy qi and pathogenic factors, deficiency and excess of the disease.

When inquiring, the doctor should be amiable, serious and conscientious, concerned with the patients and use simple language to talk with them. Only by listening to the patient's chief complaints and getting the cooperation from the patient, can the doctor obtain relatively complete and accurate information of the disease condition, thus providing reliable basis for the diagnosis and treatment of the disease.

1. Inquiry of the cold and heat

At the beginning of the disease, aversion to cold and fever may occur at the same time, mostly pertaining to exogenous exterior syndrome; serious aversion to cold and mild fever often pertains to exterior syndrome due to wind cold; serious fever and mild aversion to cold usually pertains to exterior syndrome due to wind heat.

Fever without cold accompanied by thirst, and constipation indicates excess syndrome of interior heat; fear of cold in chronic disease without fever, cold hands and feet indicate weakness of yang qi; fever in the afternoon or night in chronic disease, accompanied by reddish cheeks, night sweating, feverish sensation over the five centers (palms, soles and chest) often indicates yin deficiency and interior heat.

2. Inquiry of the sweating

Inquiry of the sweating includes quantity, time, region and nature of sweating to differentiate whether the cause is excessive pathogenic qi or insufficient healthy qi.

Anhidrosis, fever and cold mostly pertain to exterior excess syndrome; sweating, fever and aversion to wind mostly pertain to exterior deficiency syndrome; profuse sweating accompanied with high fever, polydypsia pertains to interior excess heat syndrome; profuse sweating, lassitude, weak breath, faint pulse, cold limbs are serious condition of qi collapse.

Spontaneous sweating refers to frequent sweating especially after physical movement and lacking in strength of the limbs, pertaining to qi deficiency and yang deficiency; night sweating means that sticky sweating occurs when the patient falls asleep but stops after the patient wakes up.

In addition, sweating following shivering indicates critical condition; profuse and oily sweating is called apogee sweating.

3. Inquiry of the pain

Pain is a commonly encountered subjective symptom in clinical treatment. Inquiry of the pain includes such aspects as the location, nature, degree and time of the pain.

3.1 Inquiry of the headache

Sudden attack of sharp headache often pertains to excess syndrome; frequent headache often pertains to deficiency syndrome; continuous headache accompanied with aversion to cold and fever pertains to exogenous headache; headache from time to time accompanied with dizziness usually pertains to headache due to internal injury.

3.2 Inquiry of the body pain

Body pain accompanied by cold and heat headache often pertains to exterior syndrome; body pain accompanied with fever and thirst often pertains to internal heat syndrome. Joint pain aggravated by cloudy and rainy weather or other changes of weather is called arthralgia syndrome (Bi syndrome). Wandering pain pertains to wandering arthralgia (wind Bi syndrome); sharp pain with fixed location pertains to pain arthralgia (cold Bi syndrome); pain with fixed location and heavy and numb limbs pertains to fixed arthralgia (damp Bi syndrome).

Sore and weak waist, clear and profuse urination are mostly due to kidney yang deficiency; lower back pain and sourness accompanied with constipation, dark urine pertains to kidney yin deficiency; cold and painful waist like sitting in the water is mostly due to exuberant pathogenic dampness; stabbing and fixed pain of the waist difficult to turn is often due to blood stasis.

3.3 Inquiry of the chest and abdomen

The chest and abdomen are the residence of the five zang-organs and six fu-organs. Therefore, diseases of the viscera are usually reflected on the chest and abdomen.

Cold pain in the chest, cough and spitting foam are often caused by cold pathogen attacking the lung; feverish pain in the chest and polydipsia are often caused by heat pathogen attacking the lung; stabbing pain of the chest and hypochondrium is often due to blood stasis; chest pain, cough with stinking pus and blood are often due to lung abscess; chest pain, tidal fever, night sweating, dry cough with scanty sputum or bloody sputum are often due to pulmonary tuberculosis; chest pain radiating to the back, or back pain radiating to the chest is due to thoracic obstruction.

Dull abdominal pain aggravated by cold, or spitting foam, mostly pertains to cold syndrome; unpalpable abdominal pain, preference for cold and constipation, mostly pertains to excess syndrome; abdominal pain relieved by heat and pressure, or loose stool pertains to deficiency syndrome; abdominal distension and pain, foul belching and acid regurgitation are caused by retention of food; pain around the umbilicus from time to time is often due to parasitic malnutrition.

4. Inquiry of the diet and partiality

Inquiry of the diet and partiality can enable one to understand whether the states of the viscera are deficiency or excess, whether the functions of the viscera are strong or weak. For the diagnosis of diseases caused by dysfunction of the spleen and stomach, inquiry of the diet and partiality is of great significance.

Inquiry of the diet and partiality mainly includes the inquiry of appetite, quantity of intake of food, thirst, drinking of water and food partiality.

4.1 Inquiry of the appetite and quantity of intake of food

Gradual increase of the quantity of intake of food indicates gradual restoration of stomach qi; gradual decrease of the quantity of intake of food indicates weak spleen and stomach. Polyphagia and frequent eating is usually caused by exuberance of stomach fire; hunger without desire for food is often due to insufficient stomach yin. Anorexia and disliking oily and greasy food are often seen in diseases due to internal accumulation of dampness-heatheat in the liver and gallbladder or in the spleen and stomach. Addiction to foreign bodies (raw rice, soil, etc.) is commonly encountered in infantile parasitic malnutrition. Anorexia or food partiality in the gravida usually isn't a morbid but normal phenomenon.

4.2 Inquiry of the thirst and drinking of water

Thirst with much drinking of water and preference for cold drinks are signs of consumption of body fluid due to heat exuberance; thirst with preference for hot drinks but without much drinking of water is usually due to internal cold or exuberant dampness; extreme thirst with much drinking of water and excessive urination are due to consumptive thirst.

4.3 Inquiry of the taste

Bitter taste in the mouth is usually seen in syndromes due to heat exuberance of the liver and bladder; sweet; sticky and greasy taste in the mouth is often due to dampness-heat in the spleen and stomach; sour taste in the mouth is usually caused by stagnation of heat in the liver and stomach; sour and putrid taste in the mouth is usually caused by indigestion due to retention of food; salty taste in the mouth is usually due to kidney deficiency; bland taste in the mouth is usually due to deficient spleen failing to transport or internal retention of water dampness.

5. Inquiry of the urination and defecation

Inquiry of the urination and defecation includes the frequency, nature, color, odor and bloodiness of the urination and defecation.

5.1 Inquiry of the defecation

Constipation accompanied with abdominal fullness, distension and pain or fever and thirst, pertains to excess syndrome and heat syndrome; constipation due to chronic disease, aging, pregnancy or postpartum constipation is often caused by deficiency of body fluid and blood or deficiency of qi and yin. Diarrhea following abdominal pain, burning sensation of the anus, scanty and dark urination, pertain to heat diarrhea; cold abdomen and clear urine, dull abdominal pain, poor appetite, pertain to cold diarrhea; long-term diarrhea following abdominal pain before dawn is called "morning diarrhea", pertaining to kidney yang decline; clear, sour and foul loose stool, abdominal distension and pain, and tenesmus, pertain to dysentery due to dampness-heat.

5.2 Inquiry of the urination

Clear and profuse urine pertains to deficiency and cold; brownish scanty urine pertains to heat syndrome; obstructive urination with pain and turbid urine are due to dampness-heat in the bladder; frequent urination even incontinence of urine pertains to kidney deficiency or qi deficiency.

6. Inquiry of the sleep

Inquiry of the sleep helps to understand the conditions of yin and yang of the body. Insomnia, poor appetite, lassitude, palpitation, forgetfulness, pale complexion are often due to over-thinking and deficiency of the heart and spleen; dysphoria and insomnia, tidal fever and night sweating, red tongue with scanty body fluid are often due to yin deficiency and internal heat; shallow sleep or easiness to be disturbed in sleep, sore mouth and tongue, are mostly caused by exuberant heart fire; insomnia and dreaminess, headache and bitter taste in the mouth, irritability are often due to exuberant fire in the liver and gallbladder. If the patient is sleepy and the limbs feel heavy, it is mostly due to damp exuberance; tiredness and debilitation and drowsiness are often due to sufficient yang qi; postcibal somnolence is usually due to insufficient spleen qi; somnolence following disease is sign of healthy qi failing to be restored.

7. Inquiry of the menstruation and leukorrhea

Menstruation, leukorrhea, pregnancy and delivery of baby are the specific physiological phenomena of women. Abnormal conditions of them will bring on disease. For women patients, conditions of menstruation and leukorrhea should be asked detailedly.

Advanced menstruation with reddish and profuse menstrual blood is often due to blood heat; pale and scanty menstrual blood and abdominal pain relieved by pressure are often due to deficiency of qi and blood; delayed menstruation, purplish menstrual blood with blood clot and abdominal pain before menstruation are often due to blood stasis or cold syndrome; irregular menstruation, abdominal pain aggravated by pressure, or chest distension before menstruation are often due to liver qi stagnation.

Amenorrhoea accompanied with fatigue, shortness of breath and pale complexion is due to blood deficiency; amenorrhoea accompanied with mental depression, purplish and dark tongue is often due to blood deficiency. Married women who are normally healthy but suddenly suffer from amenorrhea, vomiting, partiality of food, slippery and even pulse are probably pregnant.

Profuse, loose and whitish leukorrhea is mostly due to deficiency and cold of the spleen and kidney; profuse, thick, foul and yellowish leukorrhea is often due to internal exuberance of dampness-heat; thick, sticky, foul and bloody leukorrhea is often due to damp toxin.

Pulse-taking and Palpation

Pulse-taking and palpation means that the doctor uses his or her hand to palpate, feel and press certain part of the patient's body to diagnose disease. It includes taking the pulse and palpation.

1. Pulse-taking

Pulse-taking is an important part of Chinese Medicine diagnosis, which means that the doctor diagnoses the disease by feeling the pulse. "Cunkou diagnosis" is the main pulse-taking method commonly applied at present. Pulse over cunkou is divided into three parts: cun, guan and chi, located at the shallow region of the radial artery posterior to the palm. Specifically: The part at the region of protruding bone (the styloid process of radius) is guan pulse, the part anterior the guan pulse (end of wrist) is the cun pulse, and the part posterior the guan pulse (elbow end) is the chi pulse. The index finger, middle finger and ring finger of the doctor are put on the cun pulse, guan pulse and chi pulse respectively. Both hands have three divisions of pulse, so altogether there are six divisions of pulse. The cun pulse, guan pulse and chi pulse of the left hand correspond to the heart, liver and gallbladder, kidney respectively; the cun pulse, guan pulse and chi pulse of the right hand correspond to the lung, the spleen and stomach, the life gate respectively.

During pulse diagnosis, the patient should have a rest first and then sit erect or lie in supination. The arm is put straight at the same height of the heart and the palm turns over (upward palm position). Or the patient straightens his or her hand and bends the elbow, and the forearm and palm are put toward the opposite side (elbow-bending style). The doctor first puts the middle finger on the guan pulse (styloid process of radius), then the index finger on the cun pulse anterior to guan pulse, and ring finger on the chi pulse posterior to guan pulse. The distance between every two adjacent fingers depends on the height of the patient.

When feeling the pulse, the doctor should keep his or her breath normal and calm, concentrate on the pulse, calculate the beat of the pulse according to the clock or his or her own cycle of breath (an exhalation and an inhalation is a cycle of breath) and carefully feel the changes of depth, location, frequency and speed of the pulse in order to examine the condition of the disease.

2. Palpation

Palpation means to feel or press the skin, hands and feet, abdomen and other pathological regions to detect whether the local regions are cold or warm, soft or hard as well as whether there is tenderness or lump in order to determine the location and nature of the disease.

2.1 Pressing the surface of the skin

It is mainly to differentiate whether the surface of the skin is cold or warm, dry or moist, swelling.

2.2 Pressing hands and feet

It is mainly to understand whether the hands and feet are cold or warm.

2.3 Pressing the abdomen

It is mainly to understand whether the abdomen is soft or hard as well as whether it is painful or there is nodule or lump.

Chapter Two
Basic Proper Techniques for Health Preservation of Chinese Medicine

Section 1   Acupuncture

Acupuncture is a therapeutic method to needle certain acupoints on the body with proper needles to activate the disease resistance, regulate yin and yang, qi, blood and viscera, in order to achieve the purpose of preventing diseases. Clinically, the commonly used methods include filiform-acupuncture, hydroacupuncture, ear-acupuncture, intradermal-acupuncture and electro-acupuncture. This book will mainly introduce the operation standards of filiform acupuncture.

The filiform needles are usually used in clinical treatment.

1. Applications

Acute and chronic diseases such as stroke, migraine, prosopalgia, sciatica, diaphragmatic spasm, dysmenorrhea, urticaria, cervical spondylosis, acute lumbar sprain, strain of lumbar muscles, toothache.

2. Contraindications

The patients who are fatigued, hungry or very nervous.

Acupoints on the regions with infection, scar or swelling and pain.

Patients with hemorrhagic tendency and serious edema.

Acupoints on the vertex of infants should not be needled when the fontanel is not closed.

3. Items preparation

2% iodine tincture, 75% alcohol, sterile cotton swabs, tweezers, filiform needle box, cleansing kidney basin, blanket or bath towel if necessary, pillow, screen, etc.

4. Operation methods

4.1 Inserting method

① Nailing insertion of the needle (Inserting the needle aided by the pressure of the finger of the pressing hand). Press beside the acupoint with the nail of the thumb or the index finger of the left hand, hold the needle with the right hand and keep the needle tip closely against the nail. This method is suitable for puncturing with short needles, such as Neiguan (PC 6), Zhaohai (KI 6). ② Holding insertion of the needle (Inserting the needle with the help of the puncturing and pressing hands). Hold the needle tip with sterilized dry cotton balls held by the thumb and the index finger of the left hand, keep the needle tip on the skin surface of the acupoint. Then insert the needle into the skin with both hands. This method is suitable for puncturing the region with plump muscles with long needles, such as Huantiao (GB 30), Zhibian (BL 54). ③ Relaxed insertion of the needle (Inserting the needle with the fingers stretching the skin). Stretch the skin where the acupoint is located with the thumb and the index finger of the left hand, hold the needle with the right hand and then insert it into the area between the two fingers. This method is suitable for puncturing the acupoints located on the regions with loose skin or wrinkles, such as Guanyuan (RN 4), Tianshu (ST 25) on the abdomen. ④ Lifting and pinching insertion of the needle (Inserting the needle by pinching the skin). Pinch the skin up around the acupoint with the thumb and index finger of the left hand, insert the needle into the acupoint with the right hand. This method is suitable for puncturing the acupoints where the muscles are thin, such as Yintang (EX-HN 3), Cuanzhu (BL 2).

4.2 Angle and depth of insertion

4.2.1 Angle of insertion

The angle formed by the needle and the skin surface is usually classified into three kinds: perpendicular insertion, oblique insertion, horizontal insertion. ① Perpendicular insertion. The needle is inserted perpendicularly, means that there is an angle of 90° formed between the needle and the skin surface. This method is applicable to most aupoints on the body. ② Oblique insertion. The needle is inserted obliquely to form an angle of approximately 45° between the needle and the skin surface. This method is used for needling the acupoints close to the important viscera or tissues, or the acupoints which are not suitable for perpendicular and deep insertion. ③ Horizontal insertion. The needle is inserted transversely to form an angle of about 15°-25° between the needle and the skin surface. This method is applicable to the areas where the muscle is thin.

4.2.2 Depth of needle insertion

The principle is that the arrival of qi is achieved without impairing important organs. ① Constitution. Patients with thin and delicate constitution should be performed shallow insertion; patients with fat and strong constitution should be performed deep insertion. ② Age. Infants and the aged with weak constitution should be performed shallow insertion while young and middle-aged patients should be performed deep insertion. ③ Condition of disease. Patients with yang syndrome and new attack of disease should be performed shallow insertion while patients with yin syndrome and chronic disease should be performed deep insertion. ④ Regions. Acupoints at the regions of head, face, chest and back and other regions of thin muscle should be performed shallow insertion while acupoints at the regions of four limbs, buttock, abdomen and regions of thick muscle should be performed deep insertion.

4.3 Basic manipulation techniques

4.3.1 Lifting-thrusting

After the needle is inserted to a certain depth, the needle is lifted to the shallower layer and then thrust to the deeper layer in order to strengthen the stimulus and produce sourness, numbness, distension and heaviness sensation in the local region.

4.3.2 Twirling-rotating

After the needle is inserted to the desired depth, the needle is twirled and rotated backward and forward with large amplitude. The larger amplitude and more frequent the manipulation, the stronger the stimulus. When the sensation of sourness, numbness, distension and heaviness appears around the acupoint (arrival of qi), acupuncturist may feel heaviness, tension and unsmoothness beneath the needle.

4.4 For reinforcing and reducing manipulation

Light stimulus means reinforcing while strong stimulus means reducing, mild stimulus means mild reinforcing and reducing. Reinforcing manipulation is commonly applied for deficiency syndrome while reducing manipulation is commonly applied for excess syndrome. ①Reinforcing method. Inserting the needle slowly and shallowly, lifting and thrusting gently, twirling and rotating with small amplitude, and non-twirling and non-rotating of the retained needle and kneading and pressing the needled hole after the withdrawal of the needle mean reinforcing method. It is commonly used for deficiency syndrome. ②Reducing method. Inserting the needle rapidly and deeply, lifting and thrusting heavily, twirling and rotating with large amplitude, retaining the needle for a long time and frequent twirling and rotating of the retained needle, non-pressing the needled hole when withdrawing the needle. It is commonly used for excess syndrome. ③Mild reinforcing and reducing. This method means to insert the needle at moderate depth, stimulate with moderate strength, lift and thrust as well s twirl and rotate the needle with moderate amplitude, insert and withdraw the needle evenly. It is applicable to general patients.

5. Operation steps

Step 1: Prepare all the needed materials and put beside the bed, check the name, diagnose and prescribe the acupoints, ask the patient to urinate.

Step 2: For the patient receiving acupuncture treatment for the first time, the doctor is supposed to introduce various conditions (such as sensation of sourness, distension, numbness, heaviness and possible side effects) to ease the patient's fear.

Step 3: Choose appropriate posture according to the selected acupoints. Help the patient to loose the clothes. Use pillows of different sizes to enable the patient keep balanced and comfortable posture for a long time.

Step 4: After selecting acupoints, the doctor should press the acupoint with thumb and ask the patient's feelings.

Step 5: Sterilize the area selected for needling with 2% iodine first, select proper filiform needles according to the depth of the acupoint and weight of the patient, check whether the needle handle is secure enough, and whether the needle body and needle tip are bend or with hook. The acupuncturist should sterilize his or her hands with 75% alcohol cotton balls and deiodinate the area selected for needling with 75% alcohol cotton balls.

Step 6: Insertion. The left thumb (or index finger) pushes firmly against the area close to the acupoint. Hold the needle with the right hand and the thumb, index finger and middle finger hold the handle close to the root of the needle. Insert the needle into the skin rapidly and accurately and then twirl and rotate the needle slowly. This method is suitable for the filiform needle within 1.5 cun. (If the filiform needle is over 3 cun, holding insertion of the needle is suitable: Hold the needle tip with sterilized dry cotton balls held by the thumb and index finger of the left hand, keep the needle tip on the skin surface of the acupoint. Then insert the needle into the skin with both hands and twirl and rotate the needle to deeper level).

Step 7: The arrival of qi refers to the sensation of sourness, numbness, distension and heaviness and the sensation spreading to the distance. After arrival of qi, the acupuncturist should regulate sensation by reinforcing and reducing method or retain the needles for about 10 to 20 minutes.

Step 8: During the process of needling and retention of the needles, close attention should be paid to various possible accidents such as fainting, stuck needle, bent needle, broken needle or pneumatothorax. Corresponding management should be well prepared.

Step 9: Withdrawal of the needle. Press the skin around the acupoint slightly with sterilized dry cotton balls held by the left hand, rotate the needle handle gently and lift it slowly to the subcutaneous level with the right hand, then withdraw it quickly and press the punctured acupoint with sterilized dry cotton balls to prevent bleeding. After the treatment, the acupuncturist should count the number of the needles to make sure that all the needles are withdrawn.

Step 10: After operation, the acupuncturist should help the patient put on clothes, keep the patient in proper and comfortable lying posture, make the bed, clean the materials used in the process and put them to the original place and wash the hands.

Step 11: Record the operation process, selected acupoints, time of the retention of needles, responses and effects, and ask the patient to sign his or her name.

6. Management and prevention of possible accidents

6.1 Fainting

After insertion of needles, the patient may display such manifestations as dizziness, vertigo, pallor, chest distress, nausea and vomiting, sweating and cold limbs, palpitation and shortness of breath.

6.1.1 Management

The needle should be withdrawn immediately. The acupuncturist should remove the pillow and help the patient lie down and offer him or her some warm boiled water or sweet water. The patient's condition will be improved after a short rest. In severe cases, acupoints like Shuigou (GV 26), Zusanli (ST 36), Neiguan (PC 6) can be needled and Baihui (GV 20), Qihai (RN 6) can be moxibusted to resuscitate the patient.

6.1.2 Prevention

① For patient of weak constitution for the first visit, or the aged patient, patient with unstable neurovascular function, patient with over-hunger or patient in convalescence, the posture should be lying and the manipulation should be mild. ② The consulting room should be ventilated and in winter it should be warm. ③ Pay close attention to the patient's reaction so as to notice the sign of fainting and manage as early as possible.

6.2 Hemorrhage and hematoma

It is often caused by subcutaneous hemorrhage around the area needled.

6.2.1 Management

① For spot-like bleeding, the needled hole should be sterilized with dry cotton balls. ② If the local region is cyanotic or with hematoma, press to stop bleeding or use cold compress at the early stage. Hot compress is performed at the late stage. ③ For hematoma on the head, puncture to draw the blood under sterilized condition and then perform pressure dressing.

6.2.2 Prevention

① Be familiar with the locations of the acupoints, meridians and collaterals in case of puncturing the blood vessels. ② Patients with bleeding tendency are forbidden to be applied acupuncture.

6.3 Bent needle refers to the bending of the needle in the patient's body

6.3.1 Management

When the needle is bent, manipulation should in no case be applied. If it is caused by the change of patient's position, correct the position first and then withdraw the needle. If it is seriously bent, shake the needle body gently and withdraw the needle by following the direction of bending.

6.3.2 Prevention

The force of operation should be even, the stimulation should not be strengthened suddenly, the position of the patient should be comfortable. Ask the patient to avoid moving the body at will to prevent crash or pressure from foreign object.

6.4 Stuck needle

It is a phenomenon caused by the myofiber intertwining the needle body due to intense contract of local muscle when the patient feels nervous or the needle punctures into the tendon or perform one-way manipulation of the needle.

6.4.1 Management

① For patient afraid of needling, comfort him or her patiently, and instruct the patient to have deep breath, withdraw the needle when the muscle becomes loose. ② Pluck the needle handle or massage the area around the acupoint or insert one to two other needles around the stuck needle to relieve the muscular spasm and then withdraw the needle. ③ For myofiber intertwining, rotate the needle to the opposite direction and withdraw the needle when the myofiber becomes loose.

6.4.2 Prevention

Make good explanation to the patient of first visit. The rotation should not be of big range. When checking the needles at ordinary times, remove the needles which don't meet the quality requirements.

6.5 Broken needle

It means that the needle breaks and remains in the body.

6.5.1 Management

① Ask the patient not to change his or her position to prevent the broken needle from getting deeper. ② If the broken part protrudes over the skin, it should be removed with forceps. If the broken part is not over the skin, the skin around the needle is pressed with the hand to expose the broken end which is then removed with forceps. ③ If the above two methods can't work well, take out the broken needle with surgery.

6.5.2 Prevention

① In the process of needling and remaining of the needle, don't needle the whole body of the needle into the human body (1/4 of the needle body should be exposed). ② The needles should be regularly checked according to the requirements. Remove the ones that don't meet the quality requirements. ③ In the process of twirling the needle, avoid using tense force. If stuck needle or bent needle happens, proper management should be performed in case of broken needle.

6.6 Pneumatothorax

On puncturing the acupoints on the chest and back, deep insertion may impair the lung and lead the air to enter the thoracic cavity and cause traumatic pneumothorax.

6.6.1 Management

① Report to the doctor immediately and ask the patient to rest in half-lying position. Carefully observe the change of the disease condition. ② Avoid coughing. Give antitussive treatment if necessary. ③ For severe cases, cooperate with the doctor actively for thoracocentesis decompression.

6.6.2 Prevention

① On puncturing the acupoints located on the chest, supraclavicular fossa and suprasternal fossa, strictly master the insertion angle and depth. ② For patients with asthma, senile chronic bronchitis, emphysema, the puncturing of the above locations should be performed with caution.

Section 2 Moxibustion

Moxibustion is a treatment method in which mugwort wool as the main raw material is made into moxa roll or moxa cone to be ignited and applied to certain acupoints or affected parts of the body. With the warmth and effects of the drugs and through the conduction of the meridians, the therapeutic effects of warming and dredging the meridians, harmonizing qi and blood, reducing swelling and dissipating stagnation, dispelling dampness, restoring yang and rescuing from collapse can be achieved for the purposes of the prevention of disease, preservation of health, treatment of disease and strengthening of the constitution.

Moxibustion with moxa roll

It is a technique in which pure mugwort wool (or adding other herbal medicine) is rolled into a cylindrical moxa roll to be ignited and fumed above the surface of human body.

1. Applications

Bi syndrome, spleen deficiency, cold uterus, stroke, collapse syndrome, malposition, etc. It can also be used for the prevention of disease and health preservation.

2. Contraindications

Moxibustion is not suitable for patients with excess heat syndrome, yin deficiency and internal heat.

It is inadvisable to apply moxibustion to the regions of face and large vessels.

The abdominal region and lumbosacral region of the gravida should not be performed moxibustion.

3. Items preparation

Treatment tray, moxa sticks, ignition equipment, curved tray, narrow-mouth bottle, and bath towel and screen if necessary.

4. Operation methods

Prepare the items well and bring them to the bedside, make good explanation and check again.

Keep a proper posture, expose the moxibustion site, and keep warm in winter.

Conduct corresponding moxibustion method according to the doctor's advice. ① Mild moxibustion: Ignite the moxa stick, and apply moxibustion with the ignited end about 3 cm away from the acupoint on the skin. The patient should feel warm but no scorching locally. Usually each acupoint can be performed moxibustion for 5-7 minutes until the local skin becomes reddish. ② Bird pecking moxibustion: Light one end of the moxa stick, move it up and down like a bird pecking at a distance of 2-5 cm from the moxibustion site. Each site should be moxibusted for about 5 minutes. ③ Swirling moxibustion: Burn the moxa stick at one end, move it back and forth about 3 cm away from the moxibustion site, and perform repeated moxibustion. The moxibustion is generally performed for 20-30 minutes.

5. Precautions

For the moxibustion site, it is advisable to perform moxibustion from the upper to the lower, that is, from the top of the head, chest and back to the abdomen and four limbs.

During the process of applying moxibustion, the doctor should ask the patient whether there is burning pain at any time and adjust the distance in time to prevent burns. Observe changes of the disease condition and whether there is body pain caused by postural discomfort, understand the patient's physical and psychological feelings.

During moxibustion, the doctor should promptly bounce away moxa ash into the curved tray to prevent burns on the skin and clothes.

After moxibustion is completed, the doctor should insert the moxa stick into the narrow-mouth bottle immediately to extinguish the fire. Clean the local skin of the patient, assist the patient to dress well and keep a comfortable lying position, and open windows for ventilation as appropriate.

Clean up the items, put them back to the original places, wash hands, record and sign the name.

The skin is slightly red and scorching after moxibustion, which is normal. If small blisters appear after moxibustion, they can be absorbed by themselves without treatment. If the blister is large, the doctor should use a sterile syringe to remove the liquid in the blister, cover it with sterile gauze, and keep it dry to prevent infection.

Moxibustion with moxa cone

Moxa moxibustion is a technical operation in which pure mugwort wool is kneaded into a cone shape (like the size of wheat grain or half size of the pit of Chinese date, varying in size) and placed directly or indirectly on acupoints to apply moxibustion. It can be divided into direct moxibustion and indirect moxibustion.

1. The applications are the same as those of the moxibustion with moxa roll

2. The contraindications are the same as those of the moxibustion with moxa roll

3. Items preparation

Treatment trays, moxa cones, ignition equipment, vaseline, cotton swabs, tweezers, curved tray, and if necessary, bath towel and screen. For indirect moxibustion, the doctor should prepare ginger or garlic slices, etc.

4. Operation methods

Prepare well the items, bring them to the bedside, make explanation and check the doctor's advise.

Keep a proper posture, expose the moxibustion site, and keep warm.

Conduct moxibustion according to the doctor's advice.

① Direct moxibustion (usually non-scarring moxibustion). First apply a small amount of vaseline to the moxibustion site, place the moxa cone and ignite it. When the moxa cone burns to about 2/5, or when the patient feels burning pain, the doctor should use tweezers to remove the remaining moxa cone, put it in the curved plate, replace with a new one and then perform moxibustion again. Usually each acupoint can be moxibusted for 5-7 zhuang.

② Indirect moxibustion (usually ginger moxibustion, garlic moxibustion, salt moxibustion or aconite-cake moxibustion). Apply some vaseline to the moxibustion site, put one piece of fresh ginger or garlic or aconite-cake (first fresh ginger or single head garlic is cut into slices about 0.6 cm thick, and the center is pierced a few holes with a needle; the aconite cake is made by mixing aconite powder with yellow rice wine, 0.6-0.9 cm thick, piercing a few holes in the center with thick needle), place the moxa cone on the top and ignite it. When the moxa cone burns out or the patient feels scorching pain, the doctor should replace it with a new cone and perform moxibustion again. Usually each acupoint can be moxibusted for 3-7 zhuang. The moxibustion continues until the local skin becomes reddish but without blisters.

5. Precautions

For the moxibustion sites, it is advisable to perform from the upper to the lower, that is, from the top of the head, chest and back to the abdomen and four limbs.

When applying moxa cone, the mugwort wool on the needle handle must be twisted tightly to prevent the moxa ash from falling off and burning the skin or clothes.

When the moxa cone is burning, the doctor should observe carefully to prevent the moxa ash from falling off and burning the skin or clothes.

The extinguished moxa cone should be put into a narrow-mouth bottle to prevent re-ignition and fire.

After moxibustion, the doctor should clean the local skin and assist the patient to dress well. Arrange bed sheets, help the patient keep a comfortable position, and open windows for ventilation as appropriate.

Clean the items and put them back to the original places, wash hands, record and sign the name.

The skin is slightly red and scorching after moxibustion, which is normal. If small blisters appear after moxibustion, they can be absorbed by themselves without treatment. If the blister is large, the doctor should use a sterile syringe to remove the liquid in the blister, cover it with sterile gauze, and keep it dry to prevent infection.

Section 3 Cupping Therapy

Cupping therapy is also known as "fire cupping" or "jar-sucking method". It is a commonly used external therapy by applying suction through various kinds of jars in which a partial vacuum has been created to attach to the surface of the skin. This technique produces local negative pressure and warming effects which will cause blood congestion and slight blood stasis at the site, so as to make the meridians unobstructed and qi and blood exuberant, stimulate the meridians and collaterals and acupoints, or draw out toxin and expel pus, and achieve corresponding therapeutic effect. It has the functions of promoting blood circulation, promoting qi flow, relieving pain, reducing swelling, dispelling masses, reducing fever, dispelling wind, dissipating cold, removing dampness and drawing out pus. It is widely used in departments of Internal Medicine, Surgery, Gynecology, Pediatrics, Orthopedics, Ophthalmology and Otorhinolaryngology.

1. Applications

Rheumatism arthralgia and various nerve paralysis.

Cold, phlegm retention, cough and asthma.

Gastric pain, abdominal pain, lower back pain, beriberi.

Ulcerated carbuncle and sore in the early stage.

2. Contraindications

Patients with acute critical illness, severe heart disease, and heart failure.

People with high skin allergies, contagious diseases, skin tumors (lumps), and skin ulcers.

Patients with coagulation disorders such as thrombocytopenic purpura and hemophilia.

Apex region of the heat, locations of the arteral pulse and varicose veins.

Schizophrenia, convulsions, highly stressful and uncooperative patients.

Regions of acute traumatic fracture, moderate and severe edema.

Patients with scrofula, hernia and active tuberculosis.

Eyes, ears, mouth, nose and other orifices.

For those who wear precision metal implants such as pacemakers, electric jars and magnetic jars are prohibited.

People who are drunk, too thin, and over-fatigued.

3. Items preparation

3.1 Preparation before operation

3.1.1 Jars

Choose the corresponding jars according to different operating parts and operating methods. Point the jar in the light to make sure that the jar is intact and free of cracks, and touch with your hands to make sure that the inside and outside of the jar mouth are smooth and free of roughness. To disinfect the jar, and the inner wall should be wiped clean. Common types of jars: Glass jar, bamboo jar and other jars.

3.1.2 Location

The appropriate operation sites should be selected according to the purpose of preventive treatment. Commonly used sites include related acupoints that have health preservation, disease prevention and treatment functions, as well as thick muscles.

3.2 Position

The patient should choose a comfortable position which can be maintained for a long time and is convenient for cupping.

3.3 Preoperative preparations and precautions

The muscles of the whole body should be kept relaxed and adequate psychological preparation should be made. The operator should pay attention to the state of the patient. If tension, fear, anxiety or muscle tension occurs, psychological decompression counseling should be performed. In severe cases, stop the operation in time.

3.4 Environment

Keep the environment clean and sanitary to avoid pollution. The temperature should be kept at about 26℃ .

3.5 Disinfection

3.5.1 Disinfection of the jars

Different disinfection methods can be used for jars of different materials and purposes.

3.5.2 Disinfection sites for operation

Generally, the sites for cupping need not be disinfected, and the skin of the operation sites should be kept clean. Use 75% alcohol or 0.5%-1% povidone-iodine (iodine) cotton balls to disinfect the operation site when applying needle-cupping method and blood-letting method.

3.5.3 Disinfection of the operator

The hands of the operator can be cleaned with soapy water, and 75% alcohol cotton balls should be used in the needle-cupping therapy and blood-letting cupping therapy.

4. Operation methods

4.1 Fire cupping

The air is discharged to form negative pressure by the heat of the flame during combustion, and suck the jar on the skin. It is the most commonly used method which can be used for general diseases.

4.2 Steaming cupping

Put water in a bamboo jar and boil, use tweezers to pick up the jar, shake off water, and quickly press it on the skin to be sucked.

4.3 Air-sucking cupping

Attach the jar to the skin, use an air suction gun to draw out the air in the jar to generate negative pressure, and then suck the jar.

4.4 Water air-sucking cupping

After the jar is sucked on the skin according to the air-sucking cupping method, inject about 3 ml of normal saline or distilled water to keep the skin in the jar moist and prevent the skin from bleeding due to excessive negative pressure.

4.5 Herbal decoction cupping

Put the prepared herbs into a bag, boil it in water to a proper concentration, and then put the bamboo jar into the herbal decoction and boil for 10-15 minutes. Apply steaming cupping to the affected area. This method is mostly used for rheumatism.

4.6 Decoction-storing cupping

There are two operation methods. One is to store a certain amount of decoction in the jar, which is about half the volume of the jar, fasten it on the operation site, suck the air in the jar and attach it to the skin according to the air-sucking cupping method. The other is to store a certain amount of decoction in the glass jar, about half the volume of the jar, and then quickly suck the skin with the jar according to fire cupping method.

4.7 Needling cupping

First, needle on the acupoint, retain the needle after manipulations of reinforcing and reducing, and then conduct fire cupping with the needling point as the center. If combined with the herbal cupping, it is called needling-herbal cupping. In the application of this method, too long and thin needle is not advisable. The body and handle of the needle out of the body should not be too long. It is mostly used for rheumatic arthralgia.

5. Operation steps

Step 1: Examine the patient carefully, confirm the clinical diagnosis, and determine the cupping method according to the condition of disease.

Step 2: The drugs and equipments to be applied should be complete, and cleaned and arranged in order.

Step 3: Operation. First, expose the selected site, approach the patient before the operation and attach the jars on the skin easily with either hand. There are generally two kinds of arrangements: ① Close-packing method. The distance between every two jars is no more than 3 cm. It is used for those who have strong constitution but with pain symptoms. It has sedative, analgesic and anti-inflammatory effects, which is also known as "stimulating method". ② Sparse-arranging method. The distance between every two jars is 3-6 cm. It is used for those who have weak constitution and symptoms of numbness, sourness and softness of the limbs. which is also known as "weak stimulating method".

Step 4: Inquiry. After performed with fire cupping, the patient should be asked frequently about his or her feelings (if a glass jar is used, the skin reaction in the jar should also be observed). If the suction force of the jar is too strong that pain occurs, a small amount of air should be put in the jar. Method: Hold the jar with left hand and tilt it slightly, press the skin of the opposite side with right finger to form a tiny gap to allow air to enter slowly, stop when the air is moderately entered, and attach the jar to the skin again. If the patient feels that the sucking force is weak, pull the jar away and perform cupping once again. If other conditions occur, they should be treated symptomatically.

Step 5: Retention time of the jars. The large jar has strong suction force, and the cupping can be performed for 5-10 minutes each time; the small jar has weak suction force and the cupping can be performed for 10-15 minutes each time. In addition, cupping should be flexibly conducted according to the patient's age, constitution, disease condition, course of disease, and the site of the cupping.

Step 6: The frequency of cupping. Once a day or every other day, generally 10 times as a course of treatment, with 3-5 days' interval between 2 courses of a treatment. Special cupping method depends on specific situation.

Step 7: Withdrawal of the jar. Hold the jar with one hand and press the skin at the mouth of the jar with the other hand. When the air enters the jar slowly (the negative pressure will decrease suddenly if the air enters too fast, and this will cause pain for the patient), the jar will fall. Do not withdraw the jar forcefully in case it will damage the skin.

Step 8: Management after the withdrawal of the jar. Generally, no treatment is required. If the jar is retained for too long, large blisters appear on the skin which can be pierced with a sterile needle and coated with Methylrosanilinium Chloride Solution to prevent infection. If the needling hole is bleeding after cupping, dry sterile cotton balls can be pressed to stop the bleeding. If local bleeding is severe, it is advisable to avoid cupping in this area next time. After the treatment, allow the patient rest for 10-20 minutes before leaving.

6. Precautions

Cupping in the areas with plump muscles and few hairs. It cannot be applied to areas with thin muscles, uneven bones and many hairs.

According to the condition of the disease and different areas, different cupping methods can be adopted, and jars (or bottles) of suitable sizes can be selected. The patient's position should be appropriate.

Be careful not to burn the skin during operation. Actions should be quick when putting the ignited cotton ball into the jar to avoid scalding the skin, or apply vaseline to the local skin, which can enhance the suction force and prevent the mouth of the jar from burning the skin. During the ignition process, if the mouth of the jar is hot, the jar should be changed; when using fire cupping method and alcohol-dripping method, prevent the burning cotton from falling; when using fire-holding method, do not knock over the lit holder; when apply steaming cupping and herbal decoction cupping, shake off the hot water and decoction in the jar to prevent scalding.

When applying needling cupping, avoid hitting deep by the needle which will cause bent needle and broken needle.

When applying blood-letting cupping method, the blood-letting tools must be strictly disinfected and the amount of bleeding should be appropriate. It is not suitable for the eye and cheek areas. Patients with weak constitution, anemia, cancer or bleeding disorders, pregnant women, and women in menstrual period should not be treated by this method.

When applying walking cupping method, the mouth of the jar should be smooth, and it should not be sucked or pulled too tightly, or pushed or pulled at the bone protrusion area to avoid skin damage.

The retention time should not be too long to avoid skin blisters and burns, and generally 10 minutes is appropriate. For burns, apply methylrosanilinium chloride solution or scald cream to prevent infection.

When withdrawing the jar, the operation should be gentle. Press the muscle at the mouth of the jar to allow air to enter, and the jar will fall. It is not allowed to lift or rotate forcibly.

After cupping, if the local blood stasis is severe or painful, it can be relieved by massage. Before the local blood stasis subsides, it is not advisable to perform cupping in this area.

If the patient feels faint, remove the jar immediately and give proper treatment.

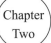

7. Reactions and management

7.1 Reactions

7.1.1 Normal reactions

Due to the negative pressure suction and pulling effect in the jar, local tissues can bulge above the surface of the jar mouth no matter what method is used to attach the jar on the treatment site. Normally, the patient may feel locally tractive, distending or feverish, tight, sensation of going-out of cool air, warm and comfortable. After the removal of jars or performance of flash cupping or walking cupping, the treatment site may appear tidal red (or purplish red) skin rash, which is the therapeutic effect after cupping therapy. After one to several days, the skin rash will subside gradually without treatment.

7.1.2 Abnormal reactions

If the patient feels abnormal tightness and pain or there is a burning sensation in the cupping area after cupping, remove the jars immediately and check whether the skin is burned or the patient is highly stressed, or the operator's technique is wrong, or the suction of the jar is too powerful, etc. Treatment should be given according to specific conditions. If cupping is not suitable on this region, other regions can be selected. If there is a lot of bleeding in the jar (the amount of bleeding exceeds the treatment requirement), after needling cupping or blood-letting cupping, remove the jar immediately and press the bleeding point with a sterile cotton ball.

7.2 Fainting

It is a special condition that occurs in cupping therapy, which is similar to fainting of needling. It often occurs during walking the jar or after cupping. Although it rarely happens, it must be prevented.

7.2.1 Symptoms of fainting of cupping

Dizziness, pale complexion, nausea and vomiting, shortness of breath, palpitation, cold extremities, accompanied by cold sweats, deep and thready pulse, declined blood pressure; in severe cases, bluish lips and nails, unconsciousness, falling to the ground, incontinence of urination and defecation, fainting pulse.

7.2.2 The cause of fainting of cupping

It occurs if cupping is performed after fasting or excessive fatigue, vomiting or sweating; or it occurs when the patient feels too nervous or has weak constitution; or the manipulation and stimulation are too strong and the cupping lasts long time, even leading to collapse syndrome and blockage syndrome.

7.2.3 Management of fainting

Ask the patient to lie supine and keep warm. For mild cases, taking warm boiled water or sugar water can help the patient quickly relieve and return to normal; for severe cases, it should be clear whether it is collapse syndrome or blockage syndrome. For collapse syndrome, warm moxibustion can be applied to consolidate collapse and restore yang and the selected acupoints include Baihui (DU 20), Zhongji (RN 3), Guanyuan (RN 4), Qihai (RN 6), Yongquan (KI 1), or salt moxibustion can be applied to Shenque (RN 8) to restore; for the patients with faint pulse, other emergency measures should be taken immediately.

7.2.4 Prevention of fainting

The operator should observe and inquiry the patient carefully. If the patient is hungry and thirsty, ask him or her to eat and then give treatment after a short period of rest; if the patient is nervous, give him or her explanation to dispel misgivings and perform cupping without his or her reluctance, and the manipulation should be gentle; during operation, if the patient feels unwell, give preventive treatment immediately.

Section 4 Scraping Therapy

Scraping therapy is to use such blunt-edge tools as horn board, porcelain spoon to repeatedly scrape a certain part of the patient's body surface to cause ecchymosis under the skin. This method allows the filthy qi of the viscera to pass through to the outside, promotes the flow of qi and blood throughout the body and eliminates the evils, thus achieving the purpose of disease prevention and treatment.

1. Applications

Painful diseases, bone and joint degenerative diseases such as cervical spondylosis.

Respiratory diseases such as cold, fever and cough.

Prevention and treatment of sub-health and chronic fatigue syndrome.

Acne, chloasma and other appearance-impaired diseases.

2. Contraindications

Patients with bleeding tendency, such as hemophilia, thrombocytopenic purpura, hemoptysis, and leukemia.

Highly neurotic, restless and uncooperative patients.

Patients with headaches, dizziness, convulsions, spasms caused by fever of the whole body.

Patients with moderate or severe heart disease or heart failure.

The region with acute traumatic fracture and patients with severe edema (edema disease).

The waist and abdomen of pregnant women and women in menstrual period.

Patients with severe skin allergies; various skin diseases and ulcers; those with damaged and ulcerated skin at the operation site; those with traumatic bone fractures; or those with varicose veins, cancer, cachexia, or inelastic skin.

Regions near large blood vessels or with superficial arterial distribution and scars.

Patients who are drunk, too thin or over-fatigued.

3. Items preparation

Treatment plate, scraping board (horn board, porcelain spoon, etc.), a small amount of water or decoction put in the treatment bowl, and bath towel, screen, etc. if necessary.

4. Operating steps

Step 1: Prepare all the items and bring them to the bedside, make an explanation and check again.

Step 2: Assist the patient to take a proper position to expose the scraping part, and keep warm in winter.

Step 3: Determine the scraping site according to the disease condition or the doctor's advice. Common sites include head, back, chest and limbs.

Step 4: Check whether the edge of the scraper is smooth to avoid scratching the skin.

Step 5: Hold the scraping board, dip it in water or decoction and scrape the skin from top to bottom on the selected part. Do not scrape back and forth in a single direction. Use force evenly and violence is prohibited.

Step 6: If scraping the back, it should start from the inside to the outside in an arc along the intercostal space on both sides of the spine, scraping for 8-10 times, each scraping about 6-15cm long.

Step 7: After scraping several times, the scraping board will become dry and should be moistened in time to continue scraping until the subcutaneous appears red or purplish red. Generally, each region should be scraped for about 20 times.

Step 8: During the scraping process, ask the patient whether there's any discomfort at any time, observe the changes of the disease condition and local skin color, and adjust the force of the operation in time.

Step 9: After scraping, clean the local skin, assist the patient to dress and place him or her in a comfortable lying position.

Step 10: Clean up the items, return to the places where they were stored, wash hands and record.

5. Precautions

Ensure ventilation of the indoor air, avoid convection wind to prevent recurrence of wind cold and aggravation of the condition.

Use uniform force during operation to avoid damaging the skin.

During the scraping process, observe the changes of disease condition at any time. If any abnormality is found, stop scraping immediately, report to and cooperate with the doctor to handle it.

After scraping, ask the patient to maintain a good mood, keep light diet and avoid cold and greasy food.

The used scraping board should be disinfected and stored for later use.

Section 5 Tuina Therapy

Tuina is applied to prevent and treat diseases through manipulations performed on certain parts of the human body to regulate the physiology and pathology of the human body.

1. Applications

Various acute and chronic diseases, such as lumbar disc herniation, cervical spondylosis, periarthritis of the shoulder, stiff neck, acute lumbar sprain, chronic lumbar muscle strain, epigastric pain, chronic diarrhea, constipation, hemiplegia, diarrhea in children, toothache.

2. Contraindications

Various bleeding diseases.

Women in menstrual period.

The waist and abdomen of pregnant women.

Skin with damage, scars, edema, etc.

3. Items preparation

Treatment tray, treatment towel, bath towel, screen.

4. Operation steps

Step 1: Explain to patients the effects and methods of Tuina for good cooperation.

Step 2: Examine the patient, confirm the diagnosis, and decide the massage techniques and location based on the condition of the disease.

Step 3: When performing waist and abdomen massage, ask the patient to urinate first.

Step 4: The patient takes a proper and comfortable position and the doctor helps loosen the patient's clothes when necessary. Keep warm in winter.

Step 5: According to the patient's symptoms, location of the disease, age and tolerance, the doctor selects appropriate techniques and stimulation intensity for massage.

Step 6: During operation, observe the patient's response to the manipulation at any time. If there is any discomfort, adjust the manipulation or stop the operation in time to prevent accidents.

Step 7: After operation, the doctor should assist the patient to put on his clothes well and keep a comfortable lying position.

Step 8: Wash hands and record if necessary.

5. The basic massage techniques

Massage is also called Tuina. There are many massage techniques in clinical practice, and some commonly-used techniques are introduced below.

5.1 Pushing manipulation (Tuifa)

Have the finger, palm or elbow exert force on a certain part and make one-way, rectilinear movements. Pushing with the finger is called finger pushing manipulation; pushing with the palm is called palm pushing manipulation and pushing with the elbow is called elbow pushing manipulation. In operating, the finger, palm and elbow should keep closely to the body surface, exertion of force should be steady at slow and even speed in order to allow heat to penetrate the skin deeply without scratching the skin.

This manipulation can be applied to all parts of the human body. It can increase muscular excitement, promote blood circulation, relax tendons and activate the meridians.

5.2 Pushing manipulation with one-finger (Yizhichan Tuifa)

Exert force on a certain site with the tip or the pulp of the finger. Relax the wrist area, drop the shoulder, hang down the elbow and suspend the wrist. Using the elbow as a pivot, sway the forearm initiatively and make it drive the wrist to sway and the thumb joint to do flexion and extension. The frequency of the manipulation is 120-160 times per minute. Pressing force, frequency, and swaying range should be even with nimble action. The patient is supposed to have heat penetrating sensation during operation.

It is often performed on the head, face, chest, abdomen and limbs.

5.3 Kneading manipulation (Roufa)

It is performed by exerting force by the major thenar, palmar base or pulp of the thumb and bringing the wrist or palm and finger to swaying slowly and softly. This manipulation should be done gently with less pressure, and its movements should be coordinative and rhythmic at a frequency of 120-160 times per minute. It is suitable for all parts of the body.

5.4 Circular rubbing manipulation (Mofa)

It is performed by fixing the palm surface or pulp of the fingers on a certain part, having the wrist together with the forearm making rhythmic and circular movements. In operation, the elbow joint should flex and extend naturally, and the wrist relaxes and the palm and fingers are straightened naturally. Action should be slow and coordinated. The frequency is about 120 circles per minute.

5.5 To-and-fro rubbing method (Cafa)

Place the major thenar, the palmar base or the minor thenar on a certain part of the body surface and do to-and-fro rubbing movements straight. In operation, extend the fingers naturally and get the whole palm and all the fingers on the treated area of the patient. The shoulder joint acts as the pivot, the upper arm moves and drives the palm to make to-and-fro or up-and-down movements. While this manipulation is operated, the action should be even and uninterrupted. Breathe naturally without holding breath. The frequency should be 100-120 times per minute. This manipulation is performed on the chest, abdomen, shoulders, waist, buttocks and limbs.

5.6 Palm-twisting manipulation (Cuofa)

The manipulation is performed by holding a certain part of the body with both palms, exerting force oppositely and doing swift, two-way twisting and kneading movements repeated. Meanwhile, both hands move up and down. In operation, the exertion of force should be symmetric, and the twisting movement should be rapid while the moving action should be slow. The force of manipulation changes from gentle to powerful, then from powerful to gentle, from slow to fast, and then from fast to slow. It is suitable for the lumbus, hypochondrium and limbs; it is generally used as an ending manipulation of Tuina treatment. It has the effects of coordinating qi and blood, relaxing tendons and dredging the meridians.

5.7 Wiping manipulation (Mafa)

This technique is done by keeping one thumb or both thumbs close to the skin and doing up-to-down and left-and-right rubbing action. In operating, exertion of force should be light but not superficial, heavy but not stuck. The manipulation is suitable for the head, face and nape. It has the effects of tranquilization, inducing resuscitation and improving eye-sight.

5.8 Vibrating manipulation (Zhenfa)

It is performed by placing the fingertips or palm on the body surface, exerting force intensively and statically with the muscles of the forearm and hand to produce vibrating movements. In manipulation, force should be concentrated on the fingertips or palm, frequency should be high and force exertion should be slightly heavy. This technique is usually operated with one hand, and operation with both hands is also applicable. It is suitable for all parts and acupoints of the body. It has the effects of eliminating phlegm, dissipating accumulation and regulating qi.

5.9 Pressing manipulation (Anfa)

It is performed by pressing the body surface with the thumb end, finger pulp, single palm or both palms and staying for a while. During the operation, the part exerting force should closely keep to the body surface of the patient without moving. The force exerted should increase from light to heavy. Sudden violent force should be avoided. Finger pressing manipulation is suitable for all acupoints of the body; palm pressing manipulation is suitable for the back and abdomen. It has the function of relaxing muscles and activating blood circulation to relive pain.

5.10 Pinching manipulation (Niefa)

It is performed by using the thumb, index finger, middle finger or thumb and the other four fingers to pinch the skin, muscles, and tendons of the affected area for squeezing. In operation, the pinching and lifting should be done one after another along a straight way without being interrupted. The movements should be even and rhythmic. This manipulation is suitable for the head, nape, shoulders, back and limbs. It has the function of relaxing the meridians and activating the collaterals, promoting qi and blood circulation.

5.11 Grasping manipulation (Nafa)

Grasping means to pinch and then lift. It is performed by using the thumb with the index and middle fingers or the other four fingers to lift and pinch certain operated parts or acupoints of the body rhythmically with opposite force. When operating, the exertion of force should be from light to strong and sudden exertion should be avoided. Operation should be even, slow and coherent. Clinically, it is often applied to the neck, nape, shoulders and limbs in combination with other manipulations. It has the function of dispelling wind and cold, relaxing tendons and dredging collaterals.

5.12 Flicking manipulation (Tanfa)

The manipulation is done by the pulp of one finger pressing firmly the other finger to make the pressed finger end to flick and hit the affected area continuously. The force exerted should be even, and the frequency is 120-160 times per minute. This manipulation is applicable to all parts of the body, especially the head, face and neck. It has the function of relaxing tendons and activating collaterals, dispelling wind and cold.

5.13 Nipping manipulation (Qiafa)

It is operated by heavily stabbing the acupoint with the nail of the thumb. This manipulation belongs to one of the manipulations inducing strong stimulation. In operating, force should be gradually given until it penetrates into the deep part, and be sure not to injure the skin. Gently kneading the local area is often applied after nipping to relieve the irritated sensation. It is often used for first aid and pain relief, which is applicable to acupoints such as Hegu (LI 4), Renzhong(GV 26), Zusanli (ST 36). It has the function of dredging blood vessels, warming and dredging meridians.

6. Precautions

The nails should be trimmed before the operation to prevent damaging the patient's skin.

The force exerted should be even, gentle, powerful and durable during operation, and sudden violent force should be avoided.

For patients with various bleeding diseases, women in menstrual period, the lumbosacral and abdominal area of the pregnant women, skin with damage or scars, this manipulation is prohibited.

Section 6 Catgut Embedding Therapy

Catgut embedding therapy is to embed catgut or biological protein thread in corresponding acupoints and specific parts under the guidance of the theories of viscera, qi and blood, and meridian system in Chinese Medicine, and utilize its continuous stimulation to the acupoints to treat diseases.

1. Applications and course of treatment

Catgut embedding therapy is commonly used to treat chronic diseases. Appropriate acupoints should be selected according to the condition of the disease.

The treatment interval and course of treatment are determined by the disease condition and the degree of absorption of the thread in the selected part. The interval is 1 week to 1 month and 3-5 times as a course of treatment depending on the disease condition.

2. Contraindications

Be cautious with catgut embedding therapy when there is bleeding tendency, mental stress, profuse sweating, tiredness or hunger.

When embedding the catgus, choose appropriate depth and angle according to different acupoints. The place of catgut embedding should not hinder the normal function and activities of the body. This therapy is prohibited for joints, facial parts and physical scars.

It is prohibited in the areas with skin diseases, ulcers, damaged skin, and tissue with scars.

Patients with diabetes, protein allergies, and other diseases that cause dysfunction of the skin and subcutaneous tissues to absorb and repair are prohibited from this therapy.

It is prohibited for the lower abdomen and lumbosacrum of pregnant women and women in menstrual period.

3. Items preparation

Suture selection. Absorbable surgical suture (length 0.5-1.0 cm).

Disposable catgut embedding needle (0.7 mm × 55 mm).

Catgut embedding kit (including scissors, treatment plate, tweezers).

Sterile gloves, masks, caps, skin disinfectants, cotton swabs, sterile dressings.

4. Preparation before operation

Absorbable surgical suture treatment: Cut the suture to segments with length of about 1 cm and use immediately after opening the package.

Acupoint selection: Select acupoints according to the patient's condition. The acupoints should be selected in muscle-rich parts. It is often applicable to the abdomen and the lower back. Be cautious with the acupoints on the face such as Fengchi (GB 20). The acupoints in the joint cavity, joints, and below the ankles and wrists as well as the acupoints in the region with blood vessels and nerve trunk such as Neiguan (PC 6) and Sanyinjiao (SP 6) are prohibited to perform this therapy. The number of acupoints selected should be controlled less than or equal to 20.

Position selection: Choose different lying positions according to the the selection of acupoints.

Environmental requirements: The operating room should be clean and sanitary, and the air should be disinfected.

Disinfection

Hand disinfection for the operator and assistant: Both hands should be disinfected according to surgical disinfection standards.

Disinfection of the instruments: The disinfection of the catgut embedding kit must meet the national hygienic standards for medical supplies and the standards for disinfection and sterilization.

Disinfection of the acupoints at the catgut embedding site: According to the operating requirements of different skin disinfectants, the operation site should be disinfected from the center to the outside circularly, with a diameter greater than 5 cm.

5. Operation steps

Step 1: Disinfection. The operator and assistant first wear masks and caps, and wash their hands in accordance with the surgical hand-washing specifications.

Step 2: Open the catgut embedding kit and surgical suture package and wear sterile gloves.

Step 3: Cut the surgical suture to segments with length of about 1.0 cm for use.

Step 4: Disposable catgut embedding needles.

Step 5: After the assistant accurately locates the selected acupoints, disinfect the local area of the patient's acupoints.

Step 6: Take a section of absorbable surgical suture with an appropriate length (about 1.0 cm) and implant it into the front end of the disposable injection needle. The end of the suture should not exceed the injection needle.

Step 7: Use the thumb and index finger of one hand to fix the acupoint to be needled, and the other hand hold the needle and insert.

Step 8: Select appropriate needling direction, penetrate into the required depth, push the needle core while withdrawing the needle tube, and embed the suture in the muscle layer or subcutaneous tissue of the acupoint.

Step 9: After removing the needle, use a sterile dry cotton swab to press the needling hole to stop bleeding, and then apply a sterile patch with a medical dressing.

6. Precautions

Strictly abide by aseptic operation. Local contact with water is prohibited within 6 hours after embedding. The wound surface should be kept dry and clean to prevent infection.

If fainting occurs, the treatment should be stopped immediately, and the fainting should be treated symptomatically.

If the suture is exposed out of the skin during the catgut embedding, it must be pulled out. Locate, disinfect and operate once again.

Strenuous exercise is prohibited within 3 days after acupoint catgut embedding to prevent swelling at the operation site.

Minimize high-protein diets such as seafood within one week after acupoint catgut embedding to prevent allergic reactions. If there is an induration reaction after embedding, apply catgut embedding therapy with caution next time.

Before embedding the catgut, the patients should be evaluated to exclude those who are not suitable for this therapy or those who do not need this therapy at present.

Chapter Three
Proper Technical Operation Specifications for Chinese Medicine Health Preservation

Chinese Medicine health preservation is about the physical and mental maintenance and protection activities from the perspective of materials and spirit. It is carried out under the guidance of Chinese Medicine theories and consciously according to the irreversible quantitative and qualitative changes of body growth and aging.

The preparation and knowledge reserves for the operators of proper technical operations of health preservation are as follows:

Information collection of the first consultation (before operation)

1. Inquiry

To understand and record the basic information of the patient, including name, age, height, weight, contact information, home address, inquire the patient's condition in detail and record the patient's chief complaints, present history, past medical history, family history, allergy history, etc. Special conditions should be recorded and marked with a red pen. Record the patient's blood pressure, heart rate, and blood sugar in detail, and mark with a red pen. If there is a history of surgery, it should be recorded in detail and marked with a red pen. Those with a history of surgery within one year should not be given treatment.

2. Inspection

Record the patient's complexion and tongue image (tongue coating, tongue texture, tooth marks, fissures, etc.) .

3. Pulse-taking and palpation

Record the patient's pulse; give necessary palpation diagnosis, record the results of palpation, tenderness and haphalgesia of the back.

4. Auscultation and olfaction

Listen to the sound and smell the odor. Record those with special conditions. Patients with lung diseases should be auscultated with a stethoscope and record the result.

5. Physical examination

According to different painful parts of the patient, do relevant physical examination and make relevant preliminary diagnosis based on the image data.

Through the collection of information, diagnosis should be made by synthesizing the four diagnostic methods.

Contraindications

To clarify the indications and contraindications of the proper techniques of Chinese Medicine health preservation, which is necessary for each operator to master. The commonly-seen contraindications are as follows:

Infectious diseases or acute or chronic infectious diseases, such as erysipelas, osteomyelitis, acute hepatitis, tuberculosis.

People with bleeding tendency, such as hemophilia or traumatic bleeding.

Patients with burns, skin disease or purulent infection in the operation area.

Patients with unclear diagnosis of acute spinal injury or with unstable spinal fractures and severe spondylolisthesis.

Patients with complete or partial rupture of tendons or ligaments.

Manipulations are prohibited for the lumbosacral area, buttocks and abdomen of pregnant women; massage of the muscles along the meridians should be prohibited or cautiously applied in women during menstrual period.

Patients with mental disease or bone fracture, joint dislocation and those who are afraid of manipulations.

Spinal massage is not applicable to abdominal distension of unknown reason, calculus of intrahepatic duct, lithiasis in urinary system or acute abdominal disease so as to avoid delaying or worsening the disease condition or causing injury.

For patients with severe local soft tissue swelling, it is necessary to find out if there are other complications, such as fractures, simple acute soft tissue injury, and manipulation should be performed with caution in the early stage.

If symptoms worsen or abnormal reactions occur after the operation, the cause should be found out before considering whether to continue the operation.

Those who suffer from severe internal disease or cannot tolerate manipulation due to old age and weak constitution; those who are too hungry, overworked, or drunk should be performed manipulation with caution.

Knowledge reserve

Those who perform proper techniques of Chinese Medicine health preservation need to have a basic Chinese Medicine knowledge reserve, among which the knowledge related to each project is the first-level and will be introduced in each project, and the second- and third-level ones are the common knowledge of the project. Detailed explanations are as follows:

1. Second-level knowledge reserve

1.1 Basic knowledge of Chinese Medicine

1.1.1 *Basic Theory of Chinese Medicine*

The philosophical basis of Chinese Medicine, including essence, qi, blood, body fluid, visceral manifestation, meridian theory, theory of constitution, etiology, pathogenesis, principles of prevention and treatment.

1.1.2 *Diagnostics of Chinese Medicine*

The basic principles of Chinese Medicine diagnostics, basic principles of Chinese Medicine diagnosis, inspection, auscultation and olfaction, inquiry, pulse-taking and palpation, syndrome differentiation with eight principles, syndrome differentiation of the nature of disease, syndrome differentiation of viscera, six-meridian syndrome differentiation, etc.

1.1.3 *Science of Meridians and Acupoints*

Overview of the meridians, overview of the acupoints, the twelve regular meridians and the acupoints, the eight extraordinary meridians and the acupoints, the extraordinary acupoints, the vertical and horizontal relationships of the meridians and collaterals, and modern study of meridians and collaterals.

1.1.4 *Science of Tuina*

The brief history of Tuina, the action mechanism of Tuina, the therapeutic principles and methods of Tuina, the commonly-used diagnostic methods, and manipulations.

1.2 Theoretical knowledge of western medicine (mainly anatomy)

1.2.1 Osteology

The composition and physiological curvature of the spine, the characteristics of each (cervical, thoracic, lumbar) vertebra, the connection between the vertebrae (the connection between the centrums, the connection between the vertebral arches).

1.2.2 Myology

The position, starting and ending points and functions of the main back muscles (trapezius, latissimus dorsi, erector spinae, etc.).

1.2.3 Nervous system

The basic functions of the nervous system, the positional relationship between spinal cord segments and vertebrae, the position and innervation area of each nerve plexus of the spinal nerve.

1.2.4 Disease

The concept, classification, and treatment method of cervical spondylosis, and the concept, classification and treatment of lumbar disc herniation.

2.Third-level knowledge reserve (synthesis of four diagnostic

methods, syndrome differentiation and treatment)

Internal Medicine of Traditional Chinese Medicine, Treatise on Cold Damage, Synopsis of the Golden Chamber, Huangdi´s Canon of Internal Medicine, Tuina Therapeutics, Acupuncture Therapeutics, Basis of Western Medicine Diagnostics, Science of Internal Medicine, etc.

Section 1 Tuina of the Meridian Sinews

Name of the project

The project of Tuina of the meridian sinews is a traditional therapy which applies Chinese Medicine massage techniques to press acupoints and specific parts along the meridian to achieve the purpose of regulating sub-health.

The function of the project

It has the function of repairing damaged tissues, clearing blocked meridians, adjusting spinal joint disorders and harmonizing spleen function.

Indications

It is applicable to the stiffness and soreness of the neck and shoulder, pain of the back, waist and lower limbs, fatigue syndrome, etc.

Standard technical operation procedures

1. Preparations

1.1 Pre-operation preparation of the operator

The operator should have good personal hygiene (including nail cutting), disinfect both hands, keep neat clothing and wear mask.

1.2 Items preparation

1 flexible operating table. ① The upper layer. 1 treatment tray, 1 scraping board put in the tray (for patient receiving scraping therapy); 1 alcohol lamp, 1 lighter, 1 hemostatic forceps, 75% alcohol cotton ball, appropriate jars; wax (for patient receiving moxibustion with wax), appropriate amount of moxa sticks (for patient receiving moxibustion treatment). ② The lower layer. 1 bed sheet, 2 towels (30 cm × 70 cm), 1 bath towel, health-preserving clothes.

1.3 Preparation of the patient

Put on health-preserving clothes and lay prone on the treatment bed.

2. Operation

Operate each technique for 3 times if there's no special instruction.

Step 1: Push the governor vessel, bladder meridian and gallbladder meridian and perform separating and pushing manipulation on the back. With the governor vessel as the midline, both hands push from the cervical spine to the lumbar spine in one direction, using the same method on the bladder meridian and gallbladder meridian. (5 minutes)

Step 2: Press and knead the bladder meridian, erector spinae and trapezius, and perform grasping and kneading manipulations on the lower legs. The main manipulations include kneading method by overlapping roots of the two palms and kneading method of the forearms. (5 minutes)

Step 3: Perform rolling manipulation from the supraspinatus to the medial side of the scapula by the small thenar, and perform rolling manipulation below the scapula by the forearm. Ask the patient about the tolerance of manipulation and adjust the strength. (5 minutes)

Step 4: Point-press Jiaji (EX-B2) and other acupoints on the back, including Jianjing (GB 21), Feishu (BL 13), Xinshu (BL 15) and other Back-Shu acupoints of the five zang-organs . Both thumbs perform point-pressing alternately. The frequency of point-pressing is the same as the patient's breathing rhythm. Press each acupoint for 3 seconds. (7 minutes)

Step 5: Perform flicking manipulation on the positive reaction points on the neck, shoulder and back. Relax the whole body and dredge the meridians; perform tendon-

25

regulating manipulation at the focal point. The key point is to find the positive reaction points and flick nearby muscles and soft tissues based on the chief complaints of the patient. (8 minutes)

Step 6: According to the patient's condition, choose appropriate treatment such as cupping, scraping, moxibustion with wax. (15 minutes)

Standards of working language

1. Before treatment

Hello, sir (madam)! Welcome! I'm your regulation physician. I'm very glad at your service. What we are doing today is the project of Tuina of the meridian sinews. Tuina of the meridian sinews can repair damaged tissues, dredge blocked meridians, and adjust spinal joint disorders. In addition, the Back-Shu acupoints are regulated through syndrome differentiation to achieve the purpose of reconciling and strengthening the viscera.

The treatment duration is about 60 minutes. Do you need to go to the bathroom? (No.)

Sir (madam), are the room temperature and lighting OK? You need to change into health-preserving clothes. I will help you hang your clothes. Please take a prone position on this bed.

2. Treatment

Follow the steps in the treatment combined with language art.

Do you feel uncomfortable in any way? I can give you regulation based on syndrome differentiation according to your condition.

Step 1: Push the governor vessel, bladder meridian, gallbladder meridian and perform separating and pushing manipulations on the back. First, let me relieve your muscular tension. How do you feel about the force? If you feel uncomfortable during my operation, please let me know in time.

Step 2: Press and knead the bladder meridian, erector spinae and trapezius, and perform grasping and kneading manipulations on the lower legs. Perform this pressing and kneading manipulations on the bladder meridian and erector spinae. The bladder meridian is the longest meridian in the human body. Each viscus in the human body has a Back-Shu acupoint along the first lateral line of the bladder meridian. The Back-Shu acupoints are the regions where qi of the viscera is infused on the back and waist. The Back-Shu acupoints have special relationships with the viscera and can reflect the deficiency, excess states of the viscera in clinical practice. We can regulate the whole by selecting Back-Shu acupoints based on syndrome differentiation. If the vertebral body is misaligned, the spinous process will have obvious tenderness, percussive pain or crookedness during palpation, and the soft tissues around the spinous process may have varying degrees of tension or even spasm. When palpating, it feels like a string and it is painful. Through the manipulation of tendons, it can dredge the meridians, improve local circulation and promote the repair of damaged tissues.

Step 3: Regulate the shoulder and neck. Modern people work for more time at the desk, and the shoulder and neck are the most fatigued parts.

In the early stage, there will be neck and shoulder pain, which will be relieved after rest, but long-term fatigue from work will lead to cervical spondylosis. Through professional manipulations, we can effectively prevent and treat headaches, dizziness, tinnitus, vertigo and other uncomfortable symptoms caused by cervical spondylosis.

3. Regulation

3.1 Moxibustion with wax

Sir (madam), the Tuina of meridian sinews has been completed. According to your condition, you are yang-deficient constitution for which the therapy of moxibustion with wax is suitable. In this therapy, it skillfully combines the Chinese medicine of Pain-Relieving Powder with heated paraffin wax. Thus it has multiple functions of invigorating blood circulation, relieving pain, dispelling wind and cold and removing dampness, quickly warming and dredging the body's meridians, dispelling wind and cold and removing dampness, so as to achieve the purpose of quickly regulating chronic disease. Combined with Tuina of meridian sinews, it can get twice the result with half the effort.

3.2 Cupping

Sir (madam), Tuina of the meridian sinews has been completed. According to your condition, there are many nodules on the back and the meridians are blocked. I will perform cupping therapy to dredge the bladder meridian on the back and retain the jar for 10-15 minutes at the pathological site (eruption of Sha, give further explanation according to the eruption of Sha) .

3.3 Scraping

Sir (madam), Tuina of the meridian sinews has been completed. According to your condition, there are many nodules on the back and your internal heat is exuberant. I will apply scraping therapy to clear away heat and blood stasis, dredge the meridians and collaterals (eruption of Sha: Give further explanation according to the eruption of Sha).

3.4 Moxibustion

Sir (madam), Tuina of the meridian sinews has been completed. According to your condition, moxibustion therapy is suitable for you. Moxibustion has multiple effects of reinforcing yang, nourishing qi, activating blood, removing cold and dampness, which can quickly warm and dredge the meridians of the body and dispel wind, cold and damp pathogens.

4. Concluding remarks

Sir (madam), that's all for the project of Tuina of the meridian sinews. Thanks for your active cooperation.

If you have any comments and suggestions, please let us know and we will definitely improve it actively.

Precautions

Pay attention to whether the room light and temperature are suitable beforehand.

The diagnosis and treatment duration is about 60 minutes, and the manipulation period is no longer than 30 minutes; for those with a history of heart disease, cervical and lumbar surgery within 2 years, the manipulation should be gentle, and the patient's feelings should be asked to adjust the manipulation.

Be careful to wrap the patient's hair with a towel to prevent the Collateral Dredging

Oil from dripping on the hair, and protect the hair during cupping.

Ask the patient not to take a bath within 6 hours.

Final treatment

1. Patient

At the end of the treatment, the patient should be instructed to avoid cold, drink more warm boiled water, and refrain from strenuous exercise that day. After putting on the clothes, the patient should be led to the hall, rest for 5-10 minutes, drink 1 cup of warm boiled water or herbal tea.

2. Arrangement of the flexible operating table and items

Clean the flexible operating table and place it in the specified location of the treatment room.

After cupping treatment, the alcohol lamp, hemostatic forceps, cotton balls, etc. should be placed to their original positions. The cupping jars should be rinsed with clean water, soaked in disinfectant for 1 hour and then taken out to dry for later use.

After scraping treatment, clean the scraping board with running water first. If necessary, use detergent to remove oil stains and other attachments so as to be clean and pollution-free. According to the different materials of the scraping tools, choose an appropriate method for cleaning and disinfection to achieve high level of disinfection. The disinfection method and selection of disinfectants must comply with the national standards. A solution containing 500-1000 mg/L of available chlorine can be used for soaking for at least 30 minutes. Obtuse tools for pressing manipulation such as stone needle can reach a moderate level of disinfection. 75% alcohol, iodine disinfectants, chlorhexidine, quaternary ammonium salts, etc. can be used to wipe and disinfect. When the instruments are contaminated, remove the contaminants in time and then clean and disinfect. When the scraping tools are contaminated by blood or body fluid, remove the contaminants in time, use a disinfectant containing 2000-5000 mg/L of chlorine to soak for at least 30 minutes, rinse with clean water and store dry. The tools can be handed over to the disinfection supply center for cleaning, disinfection and sterilization if condition permits. The scraping board should be cleaned and disinfected with alcohol, dried and stored for later use, then placed in a clean container for dry storage. The container should be cleaned and disinfected once a week. If contaminated, it should be cleaned and disinfected at any time.

Making up the room and bed unit (bed unit generally refers to the basic items contained in a hospital bed: bed sheet, bath towel, towel, etc.) .

Emergency plan

1. Allergy to Collateral-Dredging Oil

If the patient is allergic to Collateral-Dredging Oil during the operation of cupping or scraping, stop using it immediately. If the allergy is mild, wash the affected area with warm water and continue treatment with jojoba oil; if the allergy is serious, stop treatment at once, wash the affected area with warm water and give anti-allergic treatment.

2. Blisters due to cupping

If the blisters are less than 5 mm in diameter, no special treatment should be given. Take care not to break the blisters during daily activities. If the blisters are larger than 5 mm in diameter, disinfect locally. Use acupuncture needle or syringe needle to pierce the lower end of the blisters, squeeze out the liquid with cotton swabs, disinfect the affected area with povidone iodine, and instruct the patient to protect the wound in their daily lives. And pay attention to avoid eating spicy and stimulating food.

3. Blisters due to moxibustion

For the management of blisters due to moxibustion, please refer to management of blisters due to cupping.

4. Muscular pain after the Tuina of meridian sinews

Inform the patient to apply hot compress treatment, rest appropriately and reduce irritation of the painful area recently.

Knowledge reserve (knowledge related to the procedure)

Level-1 knowledge reserve

The understanding of the holistic concept of Chinese Medicine and the importance of regulation of the back.

The running routes of the meridians on the back, locations of the Back-Shu acupoints and indications.

The search for positive reaction points and the corresponding clinical manifestations.

The symptoms of neck and shoulder diseases and the importance of treatment.

The importance of symptoms and treatment of thoracic and lumbar vertebrae.

The location and indications of Jianjing (GB 21) and Tianzong (SI 11) and the importance of these two acupoints in overall regulation.

The anatomical structure, physiological function and physiological characteristics of the spine.

The basic content of yin and yang theory and its application in Chinese Medicine.

Evaluation standards of the techniques for the operation of Tuina of the Meridian Sinews

See the table below for the evaluation standards of the techniques for the operation of Tuina of the Meridian Sinews.

Evaluation standards of the techniques for the operation of Tuina of the Meridian Sinews

Total score of the project (100 points)	Requirements	Score	Evaluation description	Deduction
Quality requirements (5 points)	Presentable appearance, elegant manner, amiable attitude, neat clothes, hand washing, mask wearing.	5	Points will be deducted as appropriate according to the completion condition.	

Total score of the project (100 points)		Requirements	Score	Evaluation description	Deduction
Pre-operation preparation (25 points)	Notification	Time required for treatment, effects, techniques, possible local symptoms, obtaining of patient's cooperation.	4	Points will be deducted as appropriate according to condition of notification.	
	Evaluation	(Four diagnostic methods) present history, past history, family history, history of allergies, pregnancy or menstrual period; skin condition of the operation region, tolerance to pain, etc.	10	Points will be deducted as appropriate according to the evaluation condition.	
	Items	1 flexible operating table. The upper layer: 1 treatment tray, 1 scraping board put in the tray (operator); 1 alcohol lamp, 1 lighter, 1 hemostatic forceps, 75% alcohol cotton balls, appropriate cupping jars; 1 portion of wax mud (for moxibustion with wax); appropriate amount of moxa sticks. The lower layer: 1 bed sheet, 2 towels (30 cm×70 cm), 1 bath towel and health-preserving clothes.	5	Points will be deducted as appropriate according to the condition of imperfect item preparation.	

Continued

Total score of the project (100 points)		Requirements	Score	Evaluation description	Deduction
Pre-operation preparation (25 points)	Patients and environment	Ask the patient about preparations before treatment, take a reasonable position, and loosen clothes. Keep the room tidy, protect privacy, keep warm and avoid convection wind.	6	3 points for each of the two items. Points will be deducted as appropriate if the answer is not perfect.	
Process of the operation (40 points)	Check the doctor's advice	Check the name and diagnosis, etc.	3	3 points will be deducted if check is not performed; points will be deducted as appropriate for incomplete contents.	
	Operation	Operate in accordance with the standard technical operating procedures (steps are attached, write the scores in detail).	25	Score according to the detailed points after the table.	
	Observation	During the treatment, ask the patient about his or her feelings; comfort level and condition of pain;observe the skin condition of the operation region.	7	7 points will be deducted for failure to communicate with the patient, and points will be deducted as appropriate for incomplete contents.	

Total score of the project (100 points)		Requirements	Score	Evaluation description	Deduction
Process of the operation (40 points)	After treatment	Ask the patient about his or her feelings and inform relevant precautions; assist the patient to take a comfortable position.	5	3 points will be deducted for failure to inform, and 2 points will be deducted for failure to arrange the patient's position.	
Post-operation (20 points)	Arrangement	Make up the bed unit, arrange things, clean and disinfect the items and put them in the original places, wash hands.	5	Points will be deducted as appropriate if the arrangement is not complete.	
	Evaluation	The operation part is accurate, the manipulation is skillful, the communication with the patient is good, and the patient feels that the expected goal is achieved.	5	Points will be deducted as appropriate if the evaluation is not complete.	
	Medical record	Detailed medical records to record treatment conditions, signature.	2	2 points will be deducted for failure to record; 1 point will be deducted for incomplete records.	

Continued

Total score of the project (100 points)		Requirements	Score	Evaluation description	Deduction
Post-operation (20 points)	Post-operation disposal	Used materials are handled in accordance with "Technical Standards for Disinfection of Medical Institutions".	8	For incorrect disposal method, 2 points will be deducted for each item.	
Theoretical questions (10 points)		Knowledge about Tuina of meridian sinews. Precautions for the operation of Tuina of meridian sinews.	10	2 points will be deducted for incomplete answer of each question; 5 points will be deducted for no answer to each question.	

Total score:

Signature of the examiner:　　　　　Assessment date:

Appendix with operation steps and scoring points:

Step 1: Push the governor vessel, bladder meridian, gallbladder meridian, and perform separating and pushing manipulations on the back. (3 points)

Step 2: Press and knead the bladder meridian, erector spinae, trapezius, and grasp the calfs. (3 points)

Step 3: Perform rolling manipulation from the supraspinatus to the medial side of the scapula by the small thenar, and perform rolling manipulation below the scapula by the forearm. (3 points)

Step 4: Point-press Jiaji (EX-B2) and other acupoints on the back. (5 points)

Step 5: Perform flicking manipulation on the reaction points on the neck, shoulder and back, and focus on the positive reaction points. (6 points)

Step 6: According to the patient's condition, choose appropriate treatment such as cupping, scraping, moxibustion with wax. (5 points)

Section 2 Spinal Regulation

Name of the project

The project of spinal regulation is a therapy to regulate the dysfunction the viscera by dredging the governor vessel, bladder meridian and digital-pressing the Back-Shu acupoints.

The function of the project

It has the function of dredging the governor vessel, improving yang, unblocking the bladder meridian, adjusting spinal joint problems, improving the functions of the spine and its surrounding muscles, rebuilding the balance of spine joints and regulating Back-Shu acupoints and visceral dysfunction through syndrome differentiation.

Indications

It is applicable to shoulder and back pain, immune dysfunction, physiological hypofunction, chronic fatigue syndrome, etc.

Standard technical operation procedures

1. Preparations

1.1 Pre-operation preparation of the operator

The operator should perform personal hygiene (including nail cutting), disinfect hands, wear neat clothes and a mask.

1.2 Items preparation

1 flexible operating table. ① The upper layer: Take a vessel with a diameter of about

30 cm and a depth of 15-20 cm, add 10 drops of vacuum essential oil, 1500 ml of warm water at a temperature of about 60℃ ; 1 bottle of collateral-dredging oil (10-30 ml). 1 treatment tray, 1 scraping board put in the tray (for the patient receiving scraping); 1 alcohol lamp, 1 lighter, 1 hemostatic forceps, 75% alcohol cotton balls, appropriate jars (for the operator); 1 portion of wax (for the patient receiving moxibustion with wax); moderate amount of moxa sticks (for the patient receiving moxibustion). ② The lower layer: 1 bed sheet, 3 towels (30 cm × 70 cm), 1 bath towel and health-preserving clothes.

1.3 Preparations for the patient

Instruct the patient to change into health-preserving clothes, lie prone on the treatment bed, expose the entire back and lumbosacral area to the position of Baliao acupoints, place the upper limbs on both sides of the body. The doctor takes a towel and presses it on the edge of the patient's waist (press 1/4 width of the towel into the clothes to prevent the treatment oil from staining the clothes), then take another towel and place it at the waist of the trousers (cover the back with this towel when applying hot compress therapy).

2. Operation

Operate each technique for 3 times if there's no special instruction.

Step 1: Apply hot compress therapy. The doctor stands on the side of the bed. After communicating with the patient, put the towel in warm water to be soaked fully, and squeeze out the excess water. After testing the water temperature with the back of the hand, the doctor should spread the towel fully, apply it to the patient's entire back and stretch the entire back along the diagonal of the towel with both palms. After stretching twice, the doctor should fold 1/4 of the towel of the upper end and lower end of the towel and then fold in half, take off the hot towel with one hand, and cover the back with the prepared towel with the other hand to keep the temperature. (1minute)

Step 2: Spread oil and soothe the whole back (soothing and relaxing massage technique). ① The doctor stands beside the head of the bed, puts an appropriate amount of Collateral-Dredging Oil on the palms, rubs the palms together (dip the palms with Collateral-Dredging Oil but avoid excessive dripping on the patient's back, hair and bed sheets), puts both palms separately on the bladder meridian on both sides of the spine.

Starting from Dazhui (DU 14), the palms fully stick to the back in the order of palm base, center of the palm, finger and fingertip, then lift away from the back in the above order (the fingertips of the remaining four fingers do not leave the back except the thumb), and then repeat the above order to stick to the back, lift away from the back until the lumbosacral area, so that the back where the palms pass through is covered with Collateral-Dredging Oil. ② Raise both hands, put the fingertips of both palms opposite each other and stick close to the back on both sides of the spine, push down horizontally from Dazhui (DU 14) to the lumbosacral region, turn palms to be parallel to the spine and pull back to the level of Dazhui (DU 14). Separate the palms to the shoulders and wrap the shoulders, lift to Fengchi (GB 20) by following the direction of the trapezius muscle, and press Fengchi (GB 20) with the middle finger.

Special prompt: If the patient's back area is large, repeat the above action once in back comfort so that the back is covered with Collateral-Dredging Oil but no excessive oil flows. (1 minute)

Step 3: Dredge the governor meridian and push Baliao acupoints. Put the thumbs of both hands adjacent to the vertical direction of the spine on the governor vessel, stick the other four fingertips outwards on the back. The thumbs start from the Dazhui (DU 14) and push the governor vessel to the lumbosacral Baliao region (push along straightly or push separately). After pushing, the back can be soothed for once or twice. (2 minutes)

Step 4: Perform the route of "8" on the governor vessel. The thumbs of both hands are placed adjacently on the governor vessel in the direction perpendicular to the spine. The thumbs alternately draw arcs along the lateral side of the spinous process to under the spinous process, and alternately push until under the fifth lumbar spinous process. (2 minutes)

Step 5: Push Jiaji (EX-B2) with thumbs. Push straightly or separately of Jiaji (EX-B2) acupoints with both thumbs. Focus on and dredge the areas with nodules or muscular band (pushing or point-pressing with the thumbs). Push to the lumbosacral area and the thumbs alternately push Baliao region in arc shape. (2 minutes)

Step 6: Push the bladder meridian with the thumbs. The operation is the same as step 5, and it is performed on the first lateral line of the bladder meridian. (2 minutes)

Step 7: Half clench the fists to dredge the bladder meridian. Half clench the fists and take the joints between the fingers as the focus point to dredge the bladder meridian on both sides of the spine. Repeatedly push where there are nodules or muscular bands. (2 minutes)

Step 8: Lift and pinch acupoints on the neck, including Dazhui (DU 14), Fengchi (GB 20) and Fengfu (DU 16). The doctor should squat on the bedside, grasp and knead the shoulders with both hands, then turn to a standing position, turn the hands, overlap the thumbs, point-press Dazhui (DU 14), wrap the shoulders with both hands, lift and pull the Jianjing (GB 21) area with the part between the thumb and the index finger, lift and pull the trapezius muscle until reaching the dorsocephalad, point-press Fengchi (GB 20) of both sides with middle fingers, and then overlap the middle fingers and point-press Fengfu (DU 16). (2 minutes)

Step 9: Pluck the shoulders with both hands to expel toxins. Push the muscles of the shoulder with the thumbs from Jianliao (SJ 14) inward to Dazhui (DU 14), and then the roots of the palms immediately push it down diagonally outward. (1 minute)

Step 10: Turn around the hands and knead the neck and shoulders. Turn back the hands, half clench the fists of both hands, focus on the joints between the fingers, lift the shoulders from Jianliao (SJ 14) to Dazhui (DU 14), and then apply manipulation to the muscles on both sides of the neck. (2 minutes)

Step 11: Knead and rotationally press Dazhui (DU 14) in Tai Chi style. Rotationally press the region of Dazhui (DU 14) with the both thumbs in Tai Chi style. (1 minute)

Step 12: Point-press Jiaji (EX-B2) within two seconds. Point-press Jiaji (EX-B2) with both thumbs, 2 seconds for each point. Soothe the back after pressing the acupoints. (2 minutes)

Step 13: Turn around the hand, pull, rub and knead the scapulae. After soothing the back for the last time in the previous step, turn the palm roots from the shoulders to the lower scapular corners of both sides, press the muscles of scapular area, and lift to the region of Dazhui (DU 14). (1 minute)

Step 14: Backhand rotationally to regulate the liver and spleen. After finishing the previous step, move downward, lift and pull the areas of Ganshu (BL 18) and Danshu (BL

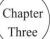

19) to Dazhui (DU 14) and move downward again, lift and pull the regions of Pishu (BL 20) and Weishu (BL 21) to Dazhui (DU 14). (1 minute)

Step 15: Double point-press Shenshu (BL 23) in saddle style. Point-press Shenshu (BL 23) with the right thumb and index finger in saddle style. (1 minute)

Step 16: Rotational manipulation for nourishing the life gate in Tai Chi style. Taking Mingmen (DU 4) as the center, both palms apply manipulations to the kidney area in Tai Chi style. (1 minute)

Step 17: Overlap the hands to dredge the triple energizer. Overlap the hands with the right hand in the lower, apply force by both hands at the same time, focus on the root of the right palm, push the governor meridian from Dazhui (DU 14) to the lumbosacral area, separate the hands from the bladder meridian on both sides to the shoulder. (2 minutes)

Step 18: Left-and-right pulling and wiping for regulating yin and yang. Put both palms on the bladder meridian on both sides of the spine, push one side from the shoulder downward to the waist and the other side from the lumbosacral area upward to the shoulder area. Manipulate both sides at the same time to regulate yin and yang for 8-10 times. (2 minutes)

Step 19: Turn around the hand, rub heat the meridians. Overlap the hands and palm-twist to heat governor meridian (with frequency of 120-160 times/min). Rub heat the kidney area and then extend upwards until the whole governor meridian has been heated. (1 minute)

Step 20: Relax the whole body to expel toxin. Soothe the back, push the trapezius of the shoulder along the direction of the arm through the lateral side of the upper arm to the medial side of the forearm, push down to the fingertips to expel toxin. (1 minute)

After the manipulation, choose the appropriate therapy according to the patient's condition, such as cupping, scraping, moxibustion with wax. (15 minutes)

Standards of working language

1. Before treatment

Hello, sir (madam)! Welcome! I'm your regulation physician. I'm very glad at your service. What we are doing today is the spinal regulation project. The spinal regulation project functions to dredge the governor meridian, lift yang qi, dredge the bladder meridian and regulate the pain and visceral diseases caused by spinal dysfunction.

The treatment duration is about 60 minutes. Do you need to go to the bathroom? (No.)

Sir (madam), are the room temperature and light OK? You need to change into health-preserving clothes. I will help you hang your clothes. Please take a prone position on this bed.

2. Treatment

Follow the steps in the treatment combined with language art.

Do you feel uncomfortable in any way? I can give you regulation based on syndrome differentiation according to your condition.

Step 1: Apply hot compress therapy. Now make a hot compress of Chinese herbal medicine on your back. Is the temperature of the medicine ok for you? (Very good.) Hot compress can relieve muscle tension. The medicinal solution and heat have a synergistic effect to dredge the meridians on the back, which paves a good way for manual treatment.

Step 2: Spread oil. Collateral-dredging oil is extracted from a variety of Chinese materia medica, with the function of dredging meridians and collaterals, removing cold and coolness.

Step 3: Dredge the governor vessel and push Baliao acupoints. What I'm doing for you now is to dredge the governor meridian. The governor vessel is the sea of yang meridians, which can stimulate and enhance yang qi, improve the symptoms of coldness, cold hands and feet caused by yang deficiency. Do you feel the force is okay?

Step 4: Perform the route of "8" on the governor vessel. In this step, I may learn the condition of your spine through the position of the spinous processes so that I can give you selective regulation later.

Step 5: Push Jiaji (EX-B2) with thumbs. This step is to dredge Jiaji (EX-B2). Jiaji (EX-B2) is closely related to the viscera and is the acupoint where the viscera are connected with the body surface of the back . Anatomically, each acupoint has a corresponding posterior branch of spinal nerve and its accompanying arteries and veins.

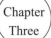
Research suggests that Jiaji (EX-B2) can regulate the function of autonomic nerves. Therefore, this acupoint is used to treat diseases related to autonomic nerve functions, such as vascular headache, acroparesthesia, autonomic dysfunction, cerebrovascular disease, hypertension.

Step 6: Push the bladder meridian with the thumbs.

Step 7: Half clench the fists to dredge the bladder meridians. Step 6 and step 7 are the techniques to dredge the bladder meridian. The bladder meridian is the longest meridian in the human body. Each viscus in the human body has a Back-Shu acupoint along the first lateral line of the bladder meridian. The Back-Shu acupoints are the regions where qi of the viscera is infused on the back and waist, and have special relationships with the viscera. They can reflect the state of the viscera in clinical practice. When these acupoints appear such abnormal reactions as nodules, muscular bands, tenderness, papules, it often reflects the abnormalities of relevant viscera. We can regulate the whole by selecting Back-Shu acupoints based on syndrome differentiation. The bladder meridian is the defensive barrier of the body. When exogenous pathogenic factors such as wind, cold, summer-heat, and dampness invade the body, disease will occur if the defensive function is poor. The good regulation of the bladder meridian can strengthen healthy qi and improve human immunity.

Step 8: Lift and pinch acupoints on the neck, including Dazhui (DU 14), Fengchi (GB 20) and Fengfu (DU 16).

Step 9: Flick the shoulders with both hands to expel toxins.

Step 10: Turn around the hands and knead the neck and shoulders.

Step 11: Knead and rotationally press Dazhui (DU 14) in Tai Chi style.

The above techniques are mainly for the regulation of the neck and shoulders. Modern people work more at desks. The neck and shoulders are the most fatigued areas. At the beginning, the neck and shoulders will be painful, which will be relieved after rest, but neglect of it will lead to cervical spondylosis. Through professional techniques, we can effectively prevent and treat headaches, dizziness, tinnitus, vertigo and other uncomfortable symptoms caused by cervical spondylosis.

Step 12: Point-press Jiaji (EX-B2) within two seconds.

Step 13: Turn around the hand, pull, rub and knead the scapulae.

Step 14: Backhand rotationally to regulate the liver and the spleen.

Step 15: Double point-press Shenshu (BL 23) in saddle style. Shenshu (BL 23) is a acupoint where the kidney essence is infused into the waist. The kidney is the root of congenital constitution. Through point-pressing the Shenshu (BL 23), the functions of strengthening the waist and invigorating the kidney can be achieved.

Step 16: Rotational manipulation for nourishing the life gate in Tai Chi style. To nourish the life gate is to nourish the kidney. According to Chinese Medicine, the kidney is the foundation of the congenital constitution. Nourishing the kidney can regulate the sourness and softness of the waist and knees, insomnia, forgetfulness and fatigue.

Step 17: Overlap the hands to dredge the triple energizer.

Step 18: Left-and-right pulling and wiping for regulating yin and yang. What I do for you now is to regulate yin and yang. According to Chinese Medicine, dynamic balance between yin and yang ensures health. This is what "yin is at peace and yang is compact" means.

Step 19: Turn around the hand, rub heat the meridians.

Step 20: Relax the whole body to expel toxin.

3.Regulation

It is the same as the "Section 1 Tuina of the meridian sinews" in this chapter.

4. Concluding remarks

Sir (madam), that's all for the project of spinal regulation. Thanks for your active cooperation. If you have any comments and suggestions, please let us know and we will definitely improve it actively.

Cautions

Pay attention to whether the lighting and temperature in the room are appropriate.

The treatment duration is about 60 minutes, and it is inadvisable for the manipulation lasts for over 30 minutes. For patients with a history of heart disease, surgery of the cervical or lumbar spine within 2 years, the manipulation should be gentle and adjusted according to the patient's feelings.

Be careful to wrap the patient's hair with a towel to prevent the oil from dripping on the hair, and protect the hair during cupping to prevent accidents.

Ask the patient not to take a bath within 6 hours.

Final treatment

1. Patient

At the end of the treatment, the patient's back should be wiped clean. Ask the patient to avoid cold, drink more warm boiled water, and refrain from strenuous exercise that day. After the patient has put on his clothes, he or she should be led to the hall, rest for 5-10 minutes and drink a cup of warm boiled water or herbal tea.

2. Arrangement of the flexible operating table and items

Clean the flexible operating table and place it in the specified location of the treatment room.

After the cupping treatment, the alcohol lamp, hemostatic forceps, cotton balls, etc. should be placed to their original positions. The cupping jars should be rinsed with clean water, soaked in disinfectant for 1 hour and then taken out to dry for later use.

After the scraping treatment, the scraping board should be cleaned, and then disinfected with alcohol and dried for later use.

Inform the visiting nurse to clean up the room.

Emergency plan

1. Allergy to Collateral-Dredging Oil

Please refer to the treatment method in the first section of this chapter "Tuina of the Meridian Sinews".

2. Blistering due to cupping

Refer to the treatment method in the first section of this chapter "Tuina of the Meridian Sinews".

3. Muscular pain after spinal regulation

Refer to the treatment method in the first section of this chapter "Tuina of the Meridian Sinews".

Knowledge reserve (knowledge related to the procedure)

Level-1 knowledge reserve

The understanding of the holistic concept of Chinese Medicine and the importance of the regulation of the back.

The running routes of the meridians on the back, location of key acupoints and indications.

The locations, meridian tropism and indications of Fengchi (GB 20) and Fengfu (DU 16).

The symptoms of neck and shoulder diseases and the importance of treatment.

The symptoms of the disease of thoracic spine and the importance of treatment.

The relationship between the liver and the spleen.

The origin of the naming, locations and indications of Shenshu (BL 23) and Mingmen (DU 4) and their importance in overall regulation.

The meaning, physiological function and physiological characteristics of the triple energizer.

The basic content of yin and yang theory and its application in Chinese Medicine.

Evaluation standards of the techniques for the operation of spinal regulation

See the table below for the evaluation standards of the techniques for the operation of spinal regulation.

Evaluation standards of the techniques for the operation of spinal regulation

Total score of the project (100 points)		Requirements	Score	Evaluation description	Deduction
Quality requirements (5 points)		Presentable appearance, elegant manner, amiable attitude, neat clothes, hand washing, mask wearing.	5	Points will be deducted as appropriate according to the completion condition.	
Pre-operation preparation (25 points)	Notification	Time required for treatment, effects, techniques, possible local symptoms, obtaining of patient's cooperation.	4	Points will be deducted as appropriate according to condition of notification.	
	Evaluation	(Four diagnostic methods) present history, past history, family history, history of allergies, pregnancy or menstrual period; skin condition of the operation region, tolerance to pain, etc.	10	Points will be deducted as appropriate according to the evaluation condition.	

Continued

Total score of the project (100 points)		Requirements	Score	Evaluation description	Deduction
Pre-operation preparation (25 points)	Items	1 flexible operating table. The upper layer: 1 utensil, 1 bottle of essential oil, 1 bottle of Collateral-Dredging Oil; 1 treatment tray, 1 scraping board put in the tray (for scraping), 1 alcohol lamp, 1 lighter, 1 hemostatic forceps, 75% alcohol cotton balls, appropriate cupping jars (for cupping); 1 portion of wax mud (for moxibustion with wax); appropriate amount of moxa sticks. The lower layer: 1 bed sheet, 3 towels (30cm×70cm), 1 bath towel and health-preserving clothes.	5	Points will be deducted as appropriate according to the condition of imperfect item preparation.	
	Patients and environment	Ask the patient about preparations before treatment, take a reasonable position, and loosen clothes. Keep the room tidy, protect privacy, keep warm and avoid convection wind.	6	3 points for each of the two items. Points will be deducted as appropriate if the answer is not perfect.	

Total score of the project (100 points)		Requirements	Score	Evaluation description	Deduction
Process of the operation (40 points)	Check the doctor's advice	Check the name and diagnosis, etc.	3	3 points will be deducted if check is not performed; points will be deducted as appropriate for incomplete contents.	
	Operation	Operate in accordance with the standard technical operating procedures (steps are attached, write the scores in detail).	25	Score according to the detailed points after the table.	
	Observation	During the treatment, ask the patient about his or her feelings; comfort level and condition of pain;observe the skin condition of the operation region.	7	7 points will be deducted for failure to communicate with the patient, and points will be deducted as appropriate for incomplete contents.	

Continued

Total score of the project (100 points)		Requirements	Score	Evaluation description	Deduction
Process of the operation (40 points)	After treatment	Ask the patient about his or her feelings and inform relevant precautions; assist the patient to take a comfortable position.	5	3 points will be deducted for failure to inform, and 2 points will be deducted for failure to arrange the patient's position.	
Post-operation (20 points)	Evaluation	The operation part is accurate, the manipulation is skillful, the communication with the patient is good, and the patient feels that the expected goal is achieved.	5	Points will be deducted as appropriate if the evaluation is not complete.	
	Medical record	Detailed medical records to record treatment conditions, signature.	2	2 points will be deducted for failure to record; 1 point will be deducted for incomplete records.	

Total score of the project (100 points)		Requirements	Score	Evaluation description	Deduction
Post-operation (20 points)	Post-operation disposal	Used materials are handled in accordance with "Technical Standards for Disinfection of Medical Institutions".	8	For incorrect disposal method, 2 points will be deducted for each item.	
Theoretical questions (10 points)		Relevant knowledge of spinal regulation. Operation precautions for spinal regulation.	10	2 points will be deducted for incomplete answer of each question; 5 points will be deducted for no answer to each question.	

Total score:

Signature of the examiner: Assessment date:

Appendix with operation steps and scoring points:

Step 1: Apply hot compress therapy. (1 point)

Step 2: Spread oil and soothe the whole back. (1 point)

Step 3: Dredge the governor meridian and push Baliao acupoints. (1 point)

Step 4: Perform the route of "8" on the governor vessel. (1 point)

Step 5: Push Jiaji (EX-B2) with thumbs. (1 point)

Step 6: Push the bladder meridian with the thumbs. (1 point)

Step 7: Half clench the fists to dredge the bladder meridian. (1 point)

Step 8: Lift and pinch acupoints on the neck, including Dazhui (DU 14), Fengchi (GB 20) and Fengfu (DU 16). (1 point)

Step 9: Pluck the shoulders with both hands to expel toxins. (1 point)

Step 10: Turn around the hands and knead the neck and shoulders. (1 point)

Step 11: Knead and rotationally press Dazhui (DU 14) in Tai Chi style. (1 point)

Step 12: Point-press Jiaji (EX-B2) within two seconds. (1 point)

Step 13: Turn around the hand, pull, rub and knead the scapulae. (1 point)

Step 14: Backhand rotationally to regulate the liver and spleen. (1 point)

Step 15: Double point-press Shenshu (BL 23) in saddle style. (1 point)

Step 16: Rotational manipulation for nourishing the life gate in Tai Chi style. (1 point)

Step 17: Overlap the hands to dredge the triple energizer. (1 point)

Step 18: Left-and-right pulling and wiping for regulating yin and yang. (1 point)

Step 19 :Turn around the hand, rub heat the meridians. (1 point)

Step 20 :Relax the whole body to expel toxin. (1 point)

After the manipulation, choose the appropriate therapy according to the patient's condition, such as cupping, scraping, moxibustion with wax. (5 point)

Section 3 Chinese Medicine for Maintaining Beauty

Name of the project

The project of Chinese medicine for maintaining beauty is a therapy by applying manipulations of pressing acupoints combined with scraping with essential oil and pure Chinese herbal masks to improve complexion and skin wrinkles.

The function of the project

It has the function of dredging the facial meridians, improving facial blood circulation, brightening complexion, reducing fine wrinkles and delaying aging.

Indications

It is suitable for sallow complexion, colored patches, skin sagging and dryness, wrinkles, etc.

Contraindications

Use with caution for the person whose face is allergic to Chinese medicine.

It is prohibited for people with facial trauma or skin problems such as dermatitis and herpes.

Those who have undergone microplastic surgery within half a year such as double eyelid operation, rhinoplasty, chinplant.

Standard technical operation procedures

1. Preparations

1.1 Pre-operation preparation for the operator

The operator should perform personal hygiene (including nail cutting), disinfect hands, wear neat clothes and a mask.

1.2 Items preparation

1 flexible operating table. ① The upper layer. 1 treatment tray, 1 bottle of facial makeup remover, eye and lip makeup remover, facial cleanser, massage cream, essential oil, softening lotion or toner, essence, day or night cream and isolation cream respectively, 1 facial mask, 1 face scraping boards, appropriate amount of cotton swabs and cotton pads, 1 face towel. ② The middle layer. 1 utensil (30 cm in diameter,15-20 cm in depth), 1 bed sheet, 3 towels (30 cm × 70 cm), 1 bath towel, and health-preserving clothes. ③ The lower layer. 1 warm water bottle and 1 sewage bucket.

1.3 Preparation of the patient

Change into health-preserving clothes, lie on the beauty care bed in a supine position, fully expose the face, cover with a bath towel on the body, and then wrap the head with a towel.

2. Operation

Operate each technique for 3 times if there is no special instructions.

2.1 Clean the face (7 minutes)

Step 1: Remove makeup. Dip a cotton swab with eye and lip makeup remover to remove makeup of the eyes and lips, and use cotton swabs and facial makeup remover to remove facial makeup.

Step 2: Use a face towel to test the water temperature on the patient's forehead, and then wipe the entire face. Operation steps: For the right side, the sequence is from the eyes, eyebrows, forehead, nose, cheek, chin to the ear; change the other side of the face towel, wipe the left half of the face (the sequence is the same as that of the right side).

Step 3: Spread the facial cleanser in five-point style (ie. forehead, cheeks, nose, chin).

Step 4: Clean the face with the middle finger and ring finger if there is no special instructions. Operation steps: ① Forehead. Make a circle from the middle of the forehead to the lateral side of the temple. ② The eyes. The operation sequence: The outer canthus, lower eyelids, inner canthus, eyebrows, and temples. ③ The nose. Circle around the tip of the nose from the medial to the lateral, then point-press Yingxiang (LI 20) acupoint, lift and pull Dicang (ST 4) through Yingxiang (LI 20) to Jingming (BL 1). ④ Around the lips. Wash the skin around the lips in "C" shapes with the middle fingers of both hands alternately. ⑤ Cheeks. The cheeks are divided into three parts and operated in circles from the medial to the lateral. Three lines: Circle from Chengjiang (RN 24) to Tinghui (GB 2); circle from Dicang (ST 4) to Tinggong (SI 19) in front of the ear; circle from Yingxiang (LI 20) to Taiyang (EX-HN5). ⑥ The neck. Pull up alternately with four fingers of two hands for 3-5 times, and then wash the ears. ⑦ The end. Clean the face with a facial towel, and pat some toner or softening lotion.

2.2 Massage (16 minutes)

Spread the massage cream in five-point style, and then operate by following the steps.

Step 1: The forehead. ① Circle by middle finger and ring finger of both hands from the middle to the sides to Taiyang (EX-HN5). ② Pull and wipe the middle area of the forehead from Yintang (EX-HN 3) to anterior hairline by the junction part between the thumb and index finger of both hands. ③ The roots of the two palms alternately wipe the entire forehead. ④ The middle finger and ring finger alternately pull in the Chinese character of "川" pattern. ⑤ Pull and spread the forehead stripes with the two hands alternately in a "C" shape. ⑥ The roots of both palms press the middle area of the forehead to finish.

Step 2: The eyes. ① Massage the skin around the eyes with the middle and ring fingers of both hands from the lateral to the medial side around the eyes. ② Pull the skin of the eye area from the inner canthus of the right eye upward and laterally to the temple with four fingers of the left hand, and pull the root of the right palm to the temple. Then operate the same way on the left side. ③ The index finger and middle finger of the left hand are in the shape of scissors. Pull the skin of the eye area from the inner canthus of the right eye upward and laterally to the temple, and pull the root of the right palm to the temple. Then operate the same way on the left side. ④ The index finger and middle finger of the left hand are placed on the upper and lower eyelids on the right side respectively, and the middle and ring fingers of the right hand knead the eye bags from the lateral side to the medial side in circle to the inner canthus. ⑤ Rub two hands hot and apply heat to both eyes.

Step 3: The nose. The technique is the same as "Clean the face" in step 4.

Step 4: The lips. Point-press the acupoints around the lips, including Renzhong (DU 26), Chengjiang (RN 24), and Dicang (ST 4), and then the two middle fingers massage the skin around the lips alternately in "C" shape.

Step 5: The cheeks. ① Take the pulps of four fingers, the thenar and the interphalangeal joints respectively as the focus points, and massage the facial skin according the "three lines" during cleansing. ② Flick both cheeks with the pulps of four fingers of both hands. ③ Cover the face with both hands, first on the right side and then on the left side. ④ Lift the jaw. Use the middle and ring fingers of both hands to lift the lower jaw vertically to the top of the head, and then use both thumbs to help the lower jaw return to its original position. ⑤ Cross the five fingers of both hands and lift the face upwards diagonally from the middle to both sides from the forehead, eyes, both sides of the nose, upper lip, and lower jaw respectively. Rub both ears with the thumbs and index fingers of both hands and flick the ears to finish. ⑥ Clean the face with a facial towel and pat some smoothing toner.

2.3 Scraping therapy (15 minutes)

Step 1: Spread the essential oil. Spread the essential oil in a five-point style, and then hold the scraping board in both hands to spread the essential oil evenly on the facial skin.

Step 2: To find out nodules. Hold the scraping board by each hand to form an angle of 45° with the facial skin. Steps to find the nodules: ① Hold the scraping board with right hand and scrape between the eyebrows and forehead with a corner of the scraping board from the governor vessel to the hairline on both sides. ② Hold the scraping boards in both hands, pull Jingming (BL 1) and scrape the eyebrow bones on both sides, and scrape diagonally upward to the hairline. ③ Start scraping from the lower eyelid, and scrape through forehead and Taiyang (EX-HN 5) diagonally upward to the hairline. ④ Scrape diagonally upwards from Yingxiang (LI 20) via frontal bone (light scraping) to Tinggong (SI 19) in front of the ear. ⑤ Scrape from Yingxiang (LI 20) via the inferior of zygomatic to Tinghui (GB 2). ⑥ Scrape the nose. ⑦ Scrape from Renzhong (DU 26) via Jiache (ST 6) to the root of the ear. ⑧ Scrape from Chengjiang (RN 24) to the root of the ear. ⑨ Use the edge of the scraping board to forcefully scrape the jaw to the posterior of the ear.

Step 3: Press and knead the nodules. Hold the scraping boards with both hands to form an angle of 30° with the skin. The procedure is the same as that in Step 2. Press and knead the nodules for half a minute with a scraping board, and scrape other regions without nodules by following general steps.

Step 4: Scrape the face. Scrape the entire face with the scraping boards in both hands by following procedure in Step 2 to finish. Clean the face with a facial towel, and pat some smoothing toner.

2.4 Apply facial mask (17 minutes)

Step 1: Prepare the facial mask. Prepare Chinese medical mask with honey and purified water, mix into thin paste (to the extent that it does not dry on the face or flow downward), with 15g of Chinese medical mask, honey, and purified water respectively.

Step 2: Apply the facial mask. Spread the mask evenly on the face and remain for 15 minutes.

2.5 Relax the head, neck and shoulders while applying the mask

Step 1: The head. ① Press Shenting (DU 24) to Baihui (GV 20) on the governor meridian with the right thumb. ② Press the bladder meridians on both sides with both thumbs (the running part of the head). ③ Scratch and knead the head with the pulps of all fingers. ④ Smooth the hair with fingers. ⑤ Knock the governor vessel, bladder meridian and gallbladder meridian with empty fists. ⑥ Scratch and knead the head with the pulps of all fingers.

Step 2: The neck. ① Knead the occiput with the pulps of fingers of the right hand. ② Knead the nape ligament and Jiaji (EX-B2) with pulps of the right fingers. ③ Pull the neck to Fengchi (GB 20) with the junction part between the thumb and index finger of the right hand.

Step 3: The shoulder. ① Press the trapezius with both hands. ② Push and press the shoulders downward with both hands. ③ Press Yunmen (LU 2) with the roots of both palms. ④ Knead the upper arm with both hands. ⑤ Knock the upper arm with empty fists of both hands.

2.6 Remove the facial mask (5 minutes)

After cleansing the face with a facial towel, apply smoothing toner, emulsion, essence, eye cream, day cream, sunscreen cream.

Standards of working language

1. Before treatment

Hello, sir (madam)! Welcome! I'm your regulation physician. I'm very glad at your service. What we are doing today is the project of Chinese medicine for maintaining beauty. The project of Chinese medicine for maintaining beauty can improve facial blood circulation, regulate colored patches on the face and improve dark complexion.

The treatment duration is about 60 minutes. Do you need to go to the bathroom? (No.)

Sir (Madam), change into health-preserving clothes and take a supine position on this bed. I will wrap your head with a towel. Is the tightness ok for you? Let's get started.

2.Treatment

Follow the steps in the treatment combined with language art.

Sir (madam), I will clean your face and remove your makeup first. Is the water temperature okay? (It's OK.)

2.1 Facial massage

Facial massage can dredge the meridians, pull small facial wrinkles and lift the facial skin. ① Forehead. The techniques on the forehead can spread the forehead horizontal wrinkles and wrinkles of Chinese character "川" shape, dredge the meridians and collaterals, and improve local blood circulation. ② The eyes. The techniques on the eyes can pull the skin around the eyes upward and obliquely, spread the crow's feet wrinkles away. Press and knead the lower eyelids can improve the blood circulation of the eyes and help relieve black circles and eye bags. Heavy dark circles indicate poor sleep or kidney deficiency. Heavy eye bags indicate yang deficiency of the spleen and kidney, and insufficient qi and blood. Local eye problems can be improved by systemic regulation. Sir (madam), is the force of the technique ok? Massage on the cheeks can improve blood circulation and moisturize the skin.

2.2 Facial scraping

Sir (madam), facial scraping is a unique feature of the project of Chinese medicine for maintaining beauty. There may be a little pain during the process. There are nodules in some areas. The face will be relaxed if the nodules are kneaded to disappear. If the force is too strong, please tell me. Face is one of the holographic areas of the body, and nodules on the face also indicate problem with the corresponding viscera. Pressing and kneading the nodules on the face also has an auxiliary regulating effect on the viscera (the problems suggested by the nodules are explained to the patient). Sir (madam), there is some Sha on the forehead which will be absorbed in two days normally, so don't worry.

2.3 Facial mask

Sir (madam), this Chinese medical mask is what we have customized for the face. It is blended with honey and purified water. Honey has the effect of moisturizing the skin, and the mask has the effect of benefiting qi, nourishing blood and dredging collaterals. Sir (madam), leave the mask for 15 minutes. I will relax your head, neck and shoulders during the mask-applying time. Now it's time to remove the mask. I'll pat some toner and apply cream for you.

Sir (madam), the project of Chinese medicine for maintaining beauty has been finished. Your facial complexion is much better than before, and your skin looks more transparent. You can take a look (show her to the mirror). Chinese medicine for maintaining beauty is a weekly facial care. It is best to do once a week. You can make an appointment with us in advance before you do it next time.

3.Concluding remarks

Sir (madam), the project of Chinese medicine for maintaining beauty has been finished. Thank you for your cooperation. If you have any comments and suggestions, please let us know and we will definitely improve it actively.

Precautions

Pay attention to whether the lighting and temperature in the room are appropriate.

The force of facial scraping should be within the patient's tolerance. It should not be too heavy.

Make sure whether there are allergic symptoms on the face during the operation.

If accidentally getting the mask into the eyes, rinse it off in time.

Be sure to wrap the head and neck with a towel to prevent essential oil from staining the hair and clothes.

Final treatment

1. Patient

At the end of the treatment, the patient will be given treatment evaluation and simple health-preserving advice. At the end of the procedure, he will be asked to rest for 5-10 minutes and drink 1 cup of warm boiled water or health-preserving herbal tea.

2. Arrangement of the flexible operating table and items

Clean the flexible operating table and place it in the specified location of the treatment room.

After washing the scraping board, place it in alcohol for disinfection for later use.

Clean up the room.

Emergency plan

1. Allergic to essential oil

If the patient is allergic to essential oil on the face, stop using it immediately. For mild allergies, scrub the affected area with warm water; for severe allergies, give anti-allergic treatment.

2. Allergic to mask

If the patient is allergic to mask, stop using the Chinese medical mask immediately. For mild allergies, scrub the affected area with warm water and give the patient an explanation; for severe allergies, give anti-allergic treatment.

Knowledge reserve

1. Level-1 knowledge reserve (knowledge related to the procedure)

The holistic concept of Chinese Medicine, the relationships among the spleen, stomach and face.

The running routes of meridians on the face, location of acupoints on the face and indications, including the locations of Taiyang (EX-HN5), Jingming (BL 1), Yingxiang (LI 20), Tinggong (SI 19), Dicang (ST 4).

Knowledge of the facial holographic area and the problems indicated by facial nodules.

The composition and function of Chinese medical mask.

The running routes and function of the meridians on the head.

Symptoms and simple treatment of neck and shoulder diseases.

2. Level-2 knowledge reserve (basic knowledge)

Introduction of Chapter 1, Health care and maintaining beauty in Chapter 2, Skin beauty in Chapter 3 of Medical Cosmetology (key points).

Evaluation standards of the techniques for the operation of Chinese medicine for maintaining beauty

See the table below for the evaluation standards of the techniques for the operation of Chinese medicine for maintaining beauty.

Evaluation standards of the techniques for the operation of Chinese medicine for maintaining beauty

Total score of the project (100 points)		Requirements	Score	Evaluation description	Deduction
Quality requirements (5 points)		Presentable appearance, elegant manner, amiable attitude, neat clothes, hand washing, mask wearing.	5	Points will be deducted as appropriate according to the completion condition.	
Pre-operation preparation (25 points)	Notification	Time required for treatment, effects, techniques, possible local symptoms, obtaining of patient's cooperation.	4	Points will be deducted as appropriate according to condition of notification.	
	Evaluation	(Four diagnostic methods) present history, past history, family history, history of allergies, pregnancy or menstrual period; skin condition of the operation region, tolcrancc to pain, etc.	10	Points will be deducted as appropriate according to the evaluation condition.	

Continued

Total score of the project (100 points)		Requirements	Score	Evaluation description	Deduction
Pre-operation preparation (25 points)	Items	1 flexible operating table. The upper layer: 1 treatment tray, 1 bottle of facial makeup remover, eye and lip makeup remover, facial cleanser, massage cream, 1 bottle of essential oil, 1 facial mask, 1 bottle of softening lotion or toner, 1 bottle of essence, 1 bottle of day or night cream and isolation cream respectively, 1 face scraping board, appropriate amount of cotton swabs and makeup cotton, 1 face towel. The lower layer: One utensil (30 cm in diameter, 15-20 cm in depth), 1 bed sheet, 3 towels (30 cm×70 cm), 1 bath towel, and health-preserving clothes.	5	Points will be deducted as appropriate according to the condition of imperfect item preparation.	
	Patients and environment	Ask the patient about preparations before treatment, take a reasonable position, and loosen clothes. Keep the room tidy, protect privacy, keep warm and avoid convection wind.	6	3 points for each of the two items. Points will be deducted as appropriate if the answer is not perfect.	

Total score of the project (100 points)		Requirements	Score	Evaluation description	Deduction
Process of the operation (40 points)	Check the doctor's advice	Check the name and diagnosis, etc.	3	3 points will be deducted if check is not performed; points will be deducted as appropriate for incomplete contents.	
	Operation	Operate in accordance with the standard technical operating procedures (steps are attached, write the scores in detail).	25	Score according to the detailed points after the table.	
	Observation	During the treatment, ask the patient about his or her feelings; comfort level and condition of pain;observe the skin condition of the operation region.	7	7 points will be deducted for failure to communicate with the patient, and points will be deducted as appropriate for incomplete contents.	

Continued

Total score of the project (100 points)		Requirements	Score	Evaluation description	Deduction
Process of the operation (40 points)	After treatment	Ask the patient about his or her feelings and inform relevant precautions; assist the patient to take a comfortable position.	5	3 points will be deducted for failure to inform, and 2 points will be deducted for failure to arrange the patient's position.	
Post-operation (20 points)	Arrangement	Make up the bed unit, arrange things, clean and disinfect the items and put them in the original places, wash hands.	5	Points will be deducted as appropriate if the arrangement is not complete.	
	Evaluation	The operation part is accurate, the manipulation is skillful, the communication with the patient is good, and the patient feels that the expected goal is achieved.	5	Points will be deducted as appropriate if the evaluation is not complete.	

Total score of the project (100 points)		Requirements	Score	Evaluation description	Deduction
Post-operation (20 points)	Medical record	Detailed medical records to record treatment conditions, signature.	2	2 points will be deducted for failure to record; 1 point will be deducted for incomplete records.	
	Post-operation disposal	Used materials are handled in accordance with "Technical Standards for Disinfection of Medical Institutions".	8	For incorrect disposal method, 2 points will be deducted for each item.	
Theoretical questions (10 points)		Relevant knowledge of Chinese medicine for maintaining beauty. The role of facial scraping in Chinese medicine for maintaining beauty.	10	2 points will be deducted for incomplete answer of each question; 5 points will be deducted for no answer to each question.	

Total score:

Signature of the examiner: Assessment date:

Appendix with operation steps and scoring points：

Cleansing of the face (7 points)

Step 1: Remove makeup. (1 point)

Step 2: Use a face towel to test the water temperature on the patient's forehead, and then wipe the entire face. (1 point)

Step 3: Spread the cleanser in five-point style. (1 point)

Step 4: Cleansing of the face. (4 points)

Massage: Spread the massage cream in five-point style, and then follow the steps (5 points)

Scraping, a total of four steps (5 points)

Facial mask: Prepare and apply the facial mask (3 points)

Relax the head and neck, a total of three steps (3 points)

Remove the facial mask, a follow the instructions above (2 points)

Section 4 Regulation of the Thoroughfare Vessel, Conception Vessel and Belt Vessel

Name of the project

The regulation of the thoroughfare vessel, conception vessel and belt vessel is a method to regulate these three vessels by applying pushing, moving manipulation along the meridians combined with moxibustion therapy to regulate women's irregular menstruation, dysmenorrhea, obesity, gastrointestinal disorders and other problems.

The function of the project

Manipulations can dredge the meridians in the lumbosacral and abdomen regions to tonify kidney qi, regulate thoroughfare vessel and conception vessel, regulate the spleen and stomach. Thus it ensures sufficient source of the generation of qi and blood, harmonious state of the thoroughfare vessel, conception vessel and belt vessel and improvement of female reproductive function.

Indications

It is suitable for premature ovarian failure, irregular menstruation, dysmenorrhea, menopausal syndrome, gastrointestinal dysfunction, etc.

Standard technical operation procedures

1. Preparations

1.1 Pre-operation preparation for the operator

The operator should do personal hygiene (including nail cutting), disinfect hands, put on clothes and caps neat, and wear a mask.

1.2 Items preparation

1 flexible operating table. ① The upper layer. Take a ware with 30 cm in diameter and 15-20 cm in depth, add 10 drops of essential oil and 1500 ml of water of the temperature about 60°C; 1 bottle of Collateral-Dredging Oil (10-30 ml), 1 alcohol lamp, 1 lighter, and appropriate amount of moxa stick. ② The lower layer. 1 bed sheet, 3 towels (30 cm ×70 cm), 1 bath towel, health-preserving clothes.

1.3 Preparation of the patient

Ask the patient to change into health-preserving clothes, lie on the bed in a prone position, expose the kidney area of the back, waist to the area of Bailiao acupoints, place the upper limbs on both sides of the body. The operation needs 2 towels and presses them on the upper and lower of the clothes in the operation region so as not to stain the clothes with oil.

2.Operation

Operate each technique for 3 times if there is no special instructions.

2.1 The waist

Step 1: Apply hot compress therapy. The doctor stands on the side of the bed, communicates with the patient, puts the towel in warm water, soaks it fully, squeezes out the excess water, and tests the water temperature with the back of the hand, then folds the towel in two layers and compresses the whole kidney area and lumbosacral area, then folds the towel in half again, removes the hot towel with one hand, and covers the back with the prepared towel with the other hand to keep the temperature. (1 minute)

Step 2: Spread oil and sooth the lumbosacral area. Spread Collateral-Dredging Oil evenly on the patient's lumbosacral area. The doctor stands on the side of the bed, takes an appropriate amount of Collateral-Dredging Oil on the palms and rubs the two palms together (to the degree that the palms are spread fully with Collateral-Dredging Oil which will not drop. It cannot drop on the patient's back, hair and sheets). Spread the oil by both palms in a circular motion from the spine to both sides so that the palms pass through the lumbosacral area and spread the full area. (1 minute)

Step 3: ① Turn on Collateral-Dredging Oil, point-press Shenshu (BL 23) and Zhishi (BL 52), push the region of Baliao acupoints backhand, point-press Baliao acupoints and then soothe the lumbosacral area. ② Press the above acupoints with both thumbs, then turn around to push the region of Baliao acupoints towards the waist direction with both thumbs, and press Baliao acupoints. After each technique, soothe the lumbosacral area once. (3 minutes)

Step 4: ① Push the belt vessel with the roots of the palms for 4-5 times. After separately pushing, push backhand to detoxify. ② The roots of both palms alternately push the belt vessel from the spine to the lateral side, and then switch to the other side. Repeat the action for 3-5 times, and soothe the waist region once after each action. (2 minutes)

Step 5: Push the kidney area in the waist with the junction parts between the thumb and index finger of both hands. Separate the thumbs of both hands from the other four fingers, push and pull in the kidney area with the junction part between the thumb and index finger. The movements should be calm, gentle and even in intensity. Push back and forth for 3-5 times and soothe the waist. (3 minutes)

Step 6: Lift-pull the belt vessel with both hands alternately and then push separately to expel toxin. Lift and pull the belt vessel on the one side for 10 times alternately with both hands, do in the same on the other side, place both palms flat on the kidney area of the waist with fingertips facing outwards and the roots of the palms facing each other, separately push the belt vessel and lift and pull upward quickly. The the force is gathered to the two palms finally and it makes a crisp clapping sound. Repeat the above action for 3-5 times. Soothe the lumbosacral area. (2 minutes)

Step 7: Rub heat the kidney area and lumbosacral area and soothe, to finish the procedure. Place the hands overlapped on the skin with fingertips perpendicular to the spine. Do a quick back-and-forth rubbing of the areas of the kidney and Baliao acupoints until it is feverish (10 times), which is the end. (2 minutes)

2.2 The abdomen

Step 1: Apply hot compress therapy. The doctor stands on the side of the bed, communicates with the patient, instructs the patient to take the supine position to expose Juque (RN 14) to Zhongji (RN 3), puts a towel on the upper and lower part of the operation area, puts the towel in warm water, and fully soaks it, squeezes out the excess water, tests the water temperature with the back of the hand, folds the towel in two layers and applies hot compress therapy to the entire abdomen, folds the towel in half neatly, removes the hot towel with one hand, covers the operation region on the abdomen with the towel by the other hand to keep the temperature. (1 minute)

Step 2: Spread oil and soothe the abdominal area. The doctor stands on the side of the bed, takes an appropriate amount of Collateral-Dredging Oil on the palms, rubs the palms together (the palms of both hands are spread fully with oil which will not drop, and it will not drop on the patient's body, hair and sheets), spreads the oil on the abdomen with two hands alternately in a circle so that the abdomen where the palms pass by is covered with oil; the hands always stick to the skin during the operation. If the patient's abdominal area is large, repeat the above action once again. (1 minute)

Step 3: ① Spread the Collateral-Dredging Oil clockwise, point-press Zhongwan (RN 12), Tianshu (ST 25), Qihai (RN 6), Guanyuan (RN 4), Zhongji (RN 3), Zigong (EX-CA1) and Guilai (ST 29), and soothe the operation area. ② Take one middle finger or thumb as the focus point and point-press the above acupoint in sequence, 3-5 times for each acupoint. After each action, soothe the operation area once. (3 minutes)

Step 4: Push along the conception vessel from Juque (RN 14) to Zhongji (RN 3), and along the stomach meridian from the free edge of the 12 ribs to Guilai (ST 29) with both palms alternately. Keep the palms sticking to the operation region and alternately push along the conception vessel from Juque (RN 14) to Zhongji (RN 3) with both palms from top to bottom. The same action goes along the stomach meridian on both sides, with left first and then right and from the free edge of the 12 ribs to the Guilai (ST 29). (3 minutes)

Step 5: Knead the upper, lower, left, right and middle of the umbilicus with the center of the palm. (3 minutes)

Step 6: Lift-pull the belt vessel with two palms alternately, separately push with both hands and expel toxin backhand. Lift-pull the belt vessel on the one side for 10 times alternately with both hands, do the same on the other side, place both palms flat on the operation region on the abdomen with fingertips facing outwards and the roots of the palms facing each other, separately push the belt vessel and lift-pull quickly. The force is gathered to the two palms finally and it makes a crisp clapping sound. Soothe the abdominal area. (2 minutes)

Step 7: Pull and wipe the belt vessel with both hands for 10 times. Put each hand on either side of the waist, and then lift on both sides with relative force, pull and wipe up and down alternately. Soothe the abdomen. (3 minutes)

Step 8: Rub heat Zigong (EX-CA 1) and Shenque (RN 8), perform moxibustion on the waist or abdomen for 30 minutes according to the patient's specific condition. (30 minutes)

Standards of working language

1. Before treatment

Hello, madam! Welcome! I'm your regulation physician. I'm very glad at your service. What we are doing today is the regulation project of the thoroughfare vessel, conception vessel and belt vessel, which has the function of dredging the meridians and collaterals, regulating qi and activating blood, regulating the thoroughfare vessel and conception vessel, warming the uterus and dispelling cold. The thoroughfare vessel and conception vessel are among the eight extraordinary meridians. According to Chinese Medicine, "The thoroughfare vessel is the sea of blood and the conception vessel dominates uterus and pregnancy". These two vessels have very close relationship with menstruation, leucorrehea, pregnancy, fetus and childbirth in women. The regulation of these two vessels by applying manipulations of pushing, arc-pushing and point-pressing acupoints is applicable for the conditioning and maintenance of female physiological functions and gastrointestinal functions.

The treatment duration is about 60 minutes. Do you need to go to the bathroom? (No.)

Madam, please change into health-preserving clothes. I will help you hang the clothes. First, please take a prone position on this bed.

2. Treatment

Follow the steps in the treatment combined with language art.

2.1 The waist

Step 1: Apply hot compress therapy. Now I'll apply hot compress therapy to to your back first. Do you think the water temperature is okay (good)? Hot compress can relieve muscle tension. The synergistic effect of the Collateral-Dredging Oil and warmth can dredge the meridians of the back, which ensures good preparation for further manipulation therapy.

Step 2: Spread oil. Collateral-Dredging Oil is extracted from a variety of Chinese materia medica, with the functions of dredging meridians and collaterals, removing cold and coolness. Do you usually feel uncomfortable in your waist and are you afraid of cold? I can give you regulation based on syndrome differentiation according to your condition.

Step 3: Spread the Collateral-Dredging Oil, point-press Shenshu (BL 23) and Zhishi (BL 52), push the triangle area backhand, point-press Baliao acupoints and soothe the lumbosacral region. What I'm doing for you now is pressing the acupoints. The waist is the residence of the kidney and the kidney governs reproduction. Many symptoms of waist soreness, aversion to cold, menstrual disorders, are related to kidney dysfunction. Shenshu (BL 23) is a acupoint where the kidney essence is infused into the waist. The kidney is the congenital foundation. Point-pressing Shenshu (BL 23) has the effect of strengthening the waist and invigorating the kidney. Shenshu (BL 23) is an important acupoint for regulating kidney function. The area of Baliao acupoints is the place which reflects gynecological problems. The manipulation of this area can improve the lumbar sourness and coldness in women. Baliao acupoints are commonly used acupoints for regulating female gynecological diseases and menstrual diseases. Do you feel the strength is okay?

Step 4: Push the belt vessel with the roots of the palms for 4-5 times. After separate pushing, expel toxin backhand. The belt vessel mainly has the effects of strengthening the spleen and remove dampness, regulating menstruation and leukorrhea.

Step 5: Push the kidney area at the waist with the junction parts between the thumb and index finger of both hands. The kidney region at the waist belongs to the the running part of the bladder meridian at the waist. Pushing the bladder meridian back and forth with both hands can help promote the smoothness of the meridians at the waist, accelerate the flow of qi and blood, relieve waist pain and strain and improve kidney function.

Step 6: Lift-pull the belt vessel with both hands alternately and then push separately to expel toxin. The belt vessel mainly has the effects of strengthening the spleen and removing dampness, regulating menstruation and leukorrhea.

Step 7: Rub warm the kidney region and lumbosacral area, and soothe to finish the whole procedure. Rubbing warm the kidney region and area of Baliao acupoints can improve kidney function, with effects of warming the kidney and nourishing yang, strengthening the waist and consolidating the kidney, regulating gynecological diseases.

2.2 The abdomen

Step 1: Apply hot compress therapy. The operation is the same as that at the waist.

Step 2: Spread oil and soothe the waist area. The operation is the same as that at the waist.

Step 3: Spread Collateral-Dredging Oil clockwise, point-press Zhongwan (RN 12), Tianshu (ST 25), Qihai (RN 6), Guanyuan (RN 4), Zhongji (RN 3), Zigong (EX-CA1), Guilai (ST 29) and soothe the operation region. Pressing the acupoints can activate meridian qi of the viscera and meridians, improve visceral function, regulate gastrointestinal function, reproductive function, immune function and physiological function, etc.

Step 4: Push along the conception vessel from Juque (RN 14) to Zhongji (RN 3), and along the stomach meridian from the free edge of the 12 ribs to Guilai (ST 29) with both palms alternately. In Chinese Medicine, it is believed that the conception vessel dominates uterus and pregnancy and is the sea of yin meridians. Females belong to yin, and thus the conception vessel plays an important role in pregnancy and occurrence of menstruation. Pushing along the stomach meridian helps digestion, enhances gastric motility and improves gastric distension, stomachache and gastric acid due to poor digestive function or disorder.

Step 5: Knead the areas above, below, on the left, on the right, in the middle of the umbilicus with palms. Kneading the area above the umbilicus can promote gastrointestinal peristalsis and improve digestive function, and the representative acupoint is Zhongwan (RN 12); kneading the area under the umbilicus can regulate uterus, improve uterine cold and irregular menstruation, and the representative acupoints includes Qihai (RN 6), Guanyuan (RN 4), Shuidao (ST 28), Guilai (ST 29); kneading the left and right of the umbilicus can promote bowel motility and improve abdominal pain, diarrhea, constipation caused by dysfunction of the large intestine, and the representative acupoint is Tianshu (ST 25); kneading the middle of the umbilicus can invigorate the root, warm yang and dispel cold, improve the symptoms of aversion to cold, clear and profuse urination, enuresis, abdominal cold, fatigue, and the representative acupoint is Shenque (RN 8) .

Step 6: Lift-pull the belt vessel with two palms alternately, separately push with both hands and expel toxin backhand. The belt vessel has the effects of invigorating the spleen and removing dampness, regulating menstruation and leukorrhea. It is mainly for the treatment of dysmenorrhea, irregular menstruation, leukorrheal diseases, pelvic inflammatory disease, and has certain regulating effect on the hypertrophy and softness in the lumbosacral area.

Step 7: Pull and wipe the belt vessel with both hands for 10 times.

Step 8: Rub warm Zigong (EX-CA1) and Shenque (RN 8) with both hands, and apply moxibustion to the operation area for 30 minutes. This technique can regulate uterine cold, dysmenorrhea, irregular menstruation, aversion and intolerance to cold and gastric cold. Madam, the manipulations for regulating thoroughfare vessel and conception vessel have been completed, and the following moxibustion therapy has multiple effects of nourishing yang, benefiting qi and activating blood, fighting against inflammation, expelling wind and dampness, rapidly warming and dredging the meridians and collaterals, removing pathogenic wind, cold and damp. Moxibustion combined with manipulations can get twice the result with half the effort.

3. Concluding remarks

Madam, this is the end of the project of regulating the thoroughfare vessel, conception vessel and belt vessel. Thanks for your cooperation. If you have any comments and suggestions, please let us know and we will definitely improve it actively.

Cautions

Before the treatment, pay attention to whether the room lighting and temperature are appropriate.

The treatment duration is about 60 minutes, and it is advisable to perform the manipulations for 30 minutes. For patients with a history of heart disease, surgery of the waist or abdomen within 2 years, the manipulations should be gentle and adjusted according to the patient's feelings.

Wrap the non-exposed parts with a towel to prevent the medical oil from staining clothes.

Observe the temperature at all times when performing moxibustion to avoid scalding the patient. The temperature should be comfortable for the patient, not too high.

Final treatment

1. Patient

At the end of the treatment, the patient will be given treatment evaluation and simple health-preserving advice. At the end of the procedure, instruct the patient to rest for 5-10 minutes and drink 1 cup of warm boiled water or health-preserving herbal tea.

2. Arrangement of the flexible operating table and items

Clean the flexible operating table and place it in the specified location of the treatment room.

Tidy the room and bed unit.

Emergency plan

1. Allergy to Collateral-Dredging Oil

Refer to the treatment method in the first section of this chapter "Tuina of the Meridian Sinews".

2.Blisters due to moxibustion

Refer to the first section of this chapter "Tuina of the Meridian Sinews" for the management of blistering due to cupping.

Knowledge reserve

Level-1 knowledge reserve

The understanding of the holistic concept of Chinese medicine, the importance of regulating the thoroughfare vessel and the conception vessel.

The running routes of the thoroughfare vessel, the conception vessel and the belt vessel, the locations and indications of key acupoints.

The locations and indications of Shenshu (BL 23) and Zhishi (BL 52).

The locations and indications of important acupoints on the abdomen.

Symptoms of the diseases at the waist and abdomen and the importance of treatment.

The relationships between the thoroughfare vessel, conception vessel and female reproductive system.

Evaluation standards of the techniques for the operation of regulation of the thoroughfare vessel, conception vessel and belt vessel

See the table below for the evaluation standards of the techniques for the operation of regulation of the thoroughfare vessel, conception vessel and belt vessel.

Evaluation standards of the techniques for the operation of regulation of the thoroughfare vessel, conception vessel and belt vessel

Total score of the project (100 points)		Requirements	Score	Evaluation description	Deduction
Quality requirements (5 points)		Presentable appearance, elegant manner, amiable attitude, neat clothes, hand washing, mask wearing.	5	Points will be deducted as appropriate according to the completion condition.	
Pre-operation preparation (25 points)	Notification	Time required for treatment, effects, techniques, possible local symptoms, obtaining of patient's cooperation.	4	Points will be deducted as appropriate according to condition of notification.	
	Evaluation	(Four diagnostic methods) present history, past history, family history, history of allergies, pregnancy or menstrual period; skin condition of the operation region, tolerance to pain, etc.	10	Points will be deducted as appropriate according to the evaluation condition.	

Total score of the project (100 points)		Requirements	Score	Evaluation description	Deduction
Pre-operation preparation (25 points)	Items	1 flexible operating table. The upper layer: Take 1 utensil with a diameter of 30 cm and a depth of 15-20 cm, add 10 drops of essential oil and 1500 ml of water at a temperature of 60°C, 1 bottle of Collateral-Dredging Oil (10-30 ml), 1 alcohol lamp and 1 lighter, appropriate amount of moxa sticks. The lower layer: 1 bed sheet, 3 towels (30 cm×70 cm), 1 bath towel and health-preserving clothes.	5	Points will be deducted as appropriate according to the condition of imperfect item preparation.	
	Patients and environment	Ask the patient about preparations before treatment, take a reasonable position, and loosen clothes. Keep the room tidy, protect privacy, keep warm and avoid convection wind.	6	3 points for each of the two items. Points will be deducted as appropriate if the answer is not perfect.	

Continued

Total score of the project (100 points)		Requirements	Score	Evaluation description	Deduction
Process of the operation (40 points)	Check the doctor's advice	Check the name and diagnosis, etc.	3	3 points will be deducted if check is not performed; points will be deducted as appropriate for incomplete contents.	
	Operation	Operate in accordance with the standard technical operating procedures (steps are attached, write the scores in detail).	25	Score according to the detailed points after the table.	
	Observation	During the treatment, ask the patient about his or her feelings; comfort level and condition of pain;observe the skin condition of the operation region.	7	7 points will be deducted for failure to communicate with the patient, and points will be deducted as appropriate for incomplete contents.	

Total score of the project (100 points)		Requirements	Score	Evaluation description	Deduction
Process of the operation (40 points)	After treatment	Ask the patient about his or her feelings and inform relevant precautions; assist the patient to take a comfortable position.	5	3 points will be deducted for failure to inform, and 2 points will be deducted for failure to arrange the patient's position.	
Post-operation (20 points)	Arrangement	Make up the bed unit, arrange things, clean and disinfect the items and put them in the original places, wash hands.	5	Points will be deducted as appropriate if the arrangement is not complete.	
	Evaluation	The operation part is accurate, the manipulation is skillful, the communication with the patient is good, and the patient feels that the expected goal is achieved.	5	Points will be deducted as appropriate if the evaluation is not complete.	
	Medical record	Detailed medical records to record treatment conditions, signature.	2	2 points will be deducted for failure to record; 1 point will be deducted for incomplete records.	

Continued

Total score of the project (100 points)		Requirements	Score	Evaluation description	Deduction
Post-operation (20 points)	Post-operation disposal	Used materials are handled in accordance with "Technical Standards for Disinfection of Medical Institutions".	8	For incorrect disposal method, 2 points will be deducted for each item.	
Theoretical questions (10 points)		Relevant knowledge of the regulation of the thoroughfare vessel, conception vessel and belt vessel. Operation precautions for the regulation of the thoroughfare vessel and conception vessel.	10	2 points will be deducted for incomplete answer of each question; 5 points will be deducted for no answer to each question.	

Total score:

Signature of the examiner: Assessment date:

Appendix with operation steps and scoring points:

1.The waist

Step 1: Apply hot compress therapy. (1 point)

Step 2: Spread oil. (1 point)

Step 3: ① Spread Collateral-Dredging Oil, point-press Shenshu (BL 23) and Zhishi (BL 52), push the region of Baliao acupoints backhand, point-press Baliao acupoints and then soothe the lumbosacral area. ② Point-press the above acupoints with both thumbs, then turn around to push the region of Baliao acupoints with both thumbs alternately at the waist, and point-press Baliao acupoints. (2 points)

Step 4: ① Push the belt vessel with the roots of the palms for 4-5 times. After separately pushing, push backhand to expel toxin. ② The roots of two palms alternately push the belt vessel from the spine to the lateral side, and then switch to the other side. (2 points)

Step 5: Push the kidney area at the waist with the junction parts between the thumb and index finger of both hands. (2 points)

Step 6: Lift-pull the belt vessel with both hands alternately and then push separately to expel toxin. (2 points)

Step 7: Rub warm the kidney area and lumbosacral area and soothe to finish the procedure. (2 points)

2.The abdomen

Step 1: Apply hot compress therapy. (1 point)

Step 2: Spread oil. (1 point)

Step 3: ① Spread the Collateral-Dredging Oil clockwise, point-press Zhongwan (RN 12), Tianshu (ST 25), Qihai (RN 6), Guanyuan (RN 4), Zhongji (RN 3), Zigong (EX-CA1) and Guilai (ST 29), and soothe the operation area. ② Take the middle finger or thumb of one hand as the focus point, point-press the above acupoints in sequence. (2 points)

Step 4: Push along the conception vessel from Juque (RN 14) to Zhongji (RN 3), and along the stomach meridian from the free edge of the 12 ribs to Guilai (ST 29) with both palms alternately. (2 points)

Step 5: Knead the parts above, below, on the left, on the right and in the middle of the umbilicus with palms. (2 points)

Step 6: Lift-pull the belt vessel with two palms alternately, push separately and backhand with both hands to expel toxin. (2 points)

Step 7: Pull and wipe the belt vessel with both hands for 10 times. (1 point)

Step 8: Rub warm the Zigong (EX-CA1) and Shenque (RN 8). Apply moxibustion on the waist or abdomen for 30 minutes according to the patient's specific condition. (2 points)

Section 5 Five-Element Suspended Moxibustion

Name of the project

The five-element suspended moxibustion is based on the concept of Chinese Medicine moxibustion for disease prevention, treatment and health preservation. In this therapy, acupoints pressing with natural essential oil is applied along the conception vessel and governor vessel. With five-element umbilical drug delivery technique, it performs suspended moxibustion on the abdomen with smokeless moxa stick and suspended moxibustion tools.

The function of the project

It has the function of dredging the conception vessel and governor vessel, harmonizing yin and yang of the five zang-organs and tonifying the five zang-organs.

Indications

The constitutional partiality includes constitution with qi deficiency, constitution with yang deficiency, constitution with qi stagnation, constitution with phlegm dampness and qi deficiency of the liver, heart, spleen, lung or kidney.

Standard technical operation procedures

1. Preparations

1.1 Pre-operation preparation of the operator

The doctor should have good personal hygiene (including nail cutting), disinfect both

---

hands, keep neat clothing and wear mask.

1.2 Items preparation

1 flexible operating table. ① The upper layer. 1 suspended moxibustion device; 1 treatment tray and 1 bottle of five-element suspended moxibustion essential oil put in the tray, 2 smokeless moxa sticks, 1 alcohol lamp, 1 lighter, 1 portion of medicinal powder for umbilical treatment and 1 special umbilical paste. ② The lower layer. 1 bed sheet, 2 towels (30 cm × 70 cm), 1 bath towel, the clothes for health preservation.

1.3 Preparation of the patient

Put on health-preserving clothes, lay prone on the treatment bed, expose the entire back and lumbosacral area to the position of Baliao acupoints, and place the upper limbs on both sides of the body. The doctor takes a towel and presses it on the edge of the waistband in the vertical direction of the back (the 1/4 width of the towel is pressed inside the clothes to prevent the five-element suspended moxibustion essential oil from staining the clothes).

2. Operation

Operate each technique for 3 times if there is no special instructions.

2.1 Dredge the meridians on the back (11 minutes)

Step 1: Spread oil and soothe the waist area. ① The doctor stands on the head of the bed, takes an appropriate amount of oil on the palms, rubs the palms together (the palms are completely spread with oil which won't drop and should not drop on the patient's back, hair and sheets). Open two palms and put them on the bladder meridians besides the spine, fully stick to the back from Dazhui (DU 14) horizontally in sequence of roots of the palms, palms, fingers and fingertips, then leave the back by following the above order (the four fingertips won't leave the back except the fingertip of thumb), repeat in the above sequence to stick to the back, leave the back until the waist region, allow the back region where both palms pass through are spread with oil. ② Raise both hands, put the fingertips of both palms opposite to each other and stick close to the back on both sides of the spine, push down horizontally from Dazhui (DU 14) to the lumbosacral region, turn palms to be parallel to the spine and pull back to the level of Dazhui (DU 14). Separate the palms to the shoulders and wrap the shoulders, lift to Fengchi (GB 20) by following the direction of the trapezius, and press Fengchi (GB 20) with middle finger. If the patient's back area is large, repeat the above action once again so that the back is covered with oil but no excess oil flows.

Step 2: To dredge the governor vessel to the region of Baliao acupoints. Put the thumbs of both hands adjacent to the vertical direction of the spine on the governor vessel, stick the other four fingertips outward to the back. The thumbs start from Dazhui (DU 14) and push the governor vessel to the region of Baliao acupoints (push along straightly or push in segments). After pushing, the back can be soothed for once or twice. (1 minute)

Step 3: Push Jiaji (EX-B2) with thumbs. Push straightly or separately of Jiaji (EX-B2) on both sides with both thumbs. Focus on and dredge the areas with nodules or muscular band (pushing or point-pressing with the thumbs). Push to the lumbosacral area and the thumbs alternately push Baliao region in arc shape. (2 minutes)

Step 4: Push the bladder meridians with the thumbs. The operation is the same as that in Step 3, and it is performed on the first lateral lines of the bladder meridians. (2 minutes)

Step 5: Half clench the fists to dredge the bladder meridians. Half clench the fists and take the joints between the fingers as the focus point to dredge the bladder meridians on both sides of the spine. Repeatedly push where there are nodules or muscular bands. (1 minute)

Step 6: Knead and press Jianjing (GB 21) and Tianzong(SI 11), dredge the medial line of the scapula. Knead and press the Jianjing (GB 21) with the thumb and Tianzong (SI 11). Push along the medial line of the scapula from top to bottom with the thumb. (1 minute)

Step 7: Soothe the waist, point-press the acupoints at the waist and push the waist separately. Soothe the waist with both hands. Press the acupoints on the bladder meridians from the first to the fourth lumbar vertebra and lumbosacral region from top to bottom. (2 minutes)

Step 8: Rub heat Mingmen (DU 4). Overlap the hands and rub the waist horizontally. (1 minute)

2.2 Dredging of the abdominal meridians (9 minutes)

Step1: Spread oil. Spread the five-element suspended moxibustion essential oil evenly on the patient's abdomen. (1 minute)

Step 2: Push the conception vessel and stomach meridian. Alternately push the conception vessel, push the stomach meridians on both sides (left first and then right). (2 minutes)

Step 3: Press the acupoints. Point-press Zhongwan (RN 12), Qihai (RN 6), Guanyuan (RN 4) and Tianshu (ST 25) respectively with the middle finger. (2 minutes)

Step 4: Knead the abdomen with the root of the palm. Overlap the hands and knead and press the abdomen with the root of the palm from the parts in the middle, on the right, above, on the left, and below the umbilicus. (2 minutes)

Step 5: Pull and wipe the belt vessel. Pull and wipe the abdomen with the junction parts between the thumbs and index fingers of both hands. (2 minutes)

2.3 Abdominal moxibustion (40 minutes)

Step 1: Drug administration on the umbilical region. Fill the umbilicus with medicinal powder for umbilical therapy, and then add the five-element suspended moxibustion essential oil.

Step 2: Ignite the smokeless moxa stick. Ignite and put the smokeless moxa stick in the suspended moxibustion device and cover the lid.

Step 3: Perform suspended moxibustion. Connect the power to turn on the governor. First connect the governor with the suspended moxibustion device, and then connect to the power supply. Adjust the governor according to the patient's feelings to control the temperature of moxibustion.

Standards of working language

1. Before treatment

Hello, sir (madam)! Welcome! I'm your regulation physician. I'm very glad at your service. The project we are going to do today is the five-element suspended moxibustion. In this therapy, natural plant essential oil is applied combined with massage technique and based on the theory of umbilical drug administration to regulate drugs for the five zang-organs, and then perform suspended moxibustion with safe, convenient and smokeless moxa stick to warm and dredge meridians and collaterals, harmonize qi and blood of five zang-organs and improve the function of the five zang-organs.

The treatment duration is about 60 minutes. Do you need to go to the bathroom? (No.)

Sir (madam), are the room temperature and brightness OK? You need to take off your coat. I will help you to hang it. Please take a prone position on this bed.

2.Treatment

Follow the steps in the treatment combined with language art.

2.1 Back

Do you feel uncomfortable in any way? I can give you regulation based on syndrome differentiation according to your condition.

Step 1: Spread oil. The five-element suspended moxibustion essential oil is specifically prepared according to the different functional characteristics of the liver, heart, spleen, lung and kidney, which is highly targeted.

Step 2: To dredge the governor vessel to the region of Baliao acupoints. The governor vessel is the sea of yang meridians. Dredging the governor vessel can stimulate and promote yang qi, improve coldness, cold hands and feet caused by yang deficiency. Do you feel the strength is okay?

Step 3: Push Jiaji (EX-B2) with the thumbs. Jiaji (EX-B2) is closely related to the viscera and is the point where the viscera and the surface of the back are connected. Anatomically, each acupoint has a corresponding posterior branch of the spinal nerve and its accompanying artery and vein. Studies show that Jiaji (EX-B2) has the function of regulating autonomic nerves, so this acupoint is used to treat diseases related to the autonomic nervous function such as vascular headache, acroparesthesia, autonomic nerve dysfunction, cerebrovascular disease, hypertension.

Step 4: Push the bladder meridians with the thumbs.

Step 5: Half clench the fists to dredge the bladder meridians. Each five zang-organ or six fu-organ has a corresponding pair of Back-Shu acupoints on the bladder meridians. The Back-Shu acupoints have special relationships with the viscera. They can reflect the state of the viscera in clinical practice. When these acupoints appear such abnormal reactions as nodules, muscular bands, tenderness, papules, it often reflects the abnormalities of relevant viscera. By regulating Back-Shu acupoints according to syndrome differentiation, the purpose of overall regulation can be achieved by local regulation. The bladder meridian is the body's defensive barrier. Protection of the bladder meridian and stimulation of its defensive function can promote healthy qi and improve human immunity.

Step 6: Knead and press Jianjing (GB 21) and Tianzong (SI 11) and the medial line of the scapula. Modern people work more at desks. The neck and shoulders are the most fatigued areas. At the beginning, the neck and shoulders will be painful, which will be relieved after rest, but neglect of it will lead to cervical spondylosis. Regulation and repair of the shoulder and neck through professional Chinese Medicine techniques can effectively prevent and treat symptoms of shoulder and back pain, hand numbness, headache, dizziness and insomnia caused by cervical spondylosis.

Step 7: Soothe the waist, point-press the acupoints at the waist and push the waist separately. The waist is the residence of the kidney. In Chinese Medicine, the kidney is the foundation of the congenital constitution. Shenshu (BL 23) is an acupoint where the kidney essence is infused into the waist. Nourishing the kidney can regulate the sourness and weakness of the waist and knees, insomnia, forgetfulness, and fatigue, thereby strengthening the waist and tonifying the kidney and enhancing the reproductive function of men and women.

2.2 Dredging of the meridians on the abdomen

Step 1: Spread oil. Spread the five-element suspended moxibustion essential oil evenly on the patient's abdomen.

Step 2: Push the conception vessel and stomach meridian. The conception vessel is the sea of yin meridians, which has the function of regulating qi of yin meridians. Dredging the stomach meridian is beneficial to regulate the digestive function of gastrointestinal tract.

Step 3: Pressing the acupoints. Pressing Zhongwan (RN 12) and Tianshu (ST 25) can enhance gastrointestinal peristalsis and promote digestion. Pressing Qihai (RN 6) and Guanyuan (RN 4) has the effect of invigorating qi and consolidating the promordial qi.

Step 4: Knead the abdomen with the roots of the palms. Overlap the hands, knead and press the parts in the middle, on the left, above, on the right, and under the umbilicus respectively. Kneading and pressing the abdomen can promote gastrointestinal peristalsis, enhance digestion, and improve symptoms of abdominal pain, constipation, diarrhea caused by intestinal dysfunction. Representative acupoints include Zhongwan (RN 12) and Tianshu (ST 25).

Step 5: Pull and wipe the belt vessel. The belt vessel has the function of restraining the meridians, removing dampness and strengthening the spleen, regulating menstruation and leukorrhea. It helps to coordinate and balance the functions of the meridians and adjust the functions of the viscera.

2.3 Abdominal moxibustion

Step 1: Drug administration on the umbilical region. Shenque (RN 8) at the umbilicus serves as the gateway to the promordial spirit, so it has the effect of restoring yang and rescuing from collapse, resuscitating and recovering consciousness. Shenque (RN 8) is located in the middle of the abdomen, which is the hub of the human body and is adjacent to the stomach, large intestine, small intestine and uterus. This acupoint can strengthen the spleen and stomach, regulate the intestines and relieve diarrhea, benefit the primordial qi and consolidate the root and regulate the physiological functions. Medicinal powder for umbilical therapy and five-element suspended moxibustion essential oil can improve various diseases caused by the dysfunction of the liver, heart, spleen, lung, and kidney, such as emotional depression and hypochondriac distention and pain, irregular menstruation due to liver depression; palpitation, shortness of breath (aggravated during activity), chest tightness, spontaneous sweating, thin and weak pulse or knotted and intermittent pulse caused by insufficient heart qi; poor appetite, abdominal distension, abdominal pain and loose stools caused by deficiency of spleen qi and yang; weak breath, fatigue, asthma after a little activity, shortness of breath caused by lung qi deficiency; low disease resistance of the human body; cold limbs, fatigue, and nocturia caused by kidney yang deficiency.

Step 2: Ignite the smokeless moxa stick. Avoid smoke pollution.

Step 3: Perform suspended moxibustion. It can be raised or lowered, and the height can be adjusted according to different constitutions, heat resistance and patient's need, which is very convenient.

3. Concluding remarks

Sir (madam), this is the end of the project of the five-element suspended moxibustion. Thanks for your active cooperation. If you have any comments and suggestions, please let us know and we will improve actively.

Cautions

Before the treatment, pay attention to whether the room lighting and temperature are appropriate.

The treatment duration is about 60 minutes, and it is advisable to perform the manipulations for 20 minutes. For patients with a history of heart disease, surgery of the spinal vertebrae within 2 years, the manipulations should be gentle and adjusted according to the patient's feelings.

For female patients with long hair, pay attention to wrap the hair with a towel.

Observe the temperature at all times when performing moxibustion to avoid scalding the patient. The temperature should be comfortable for the patient, and it should not be too hot. Tell the patient that it does not mean that the higher the temperature, the better.

Ask the patient not to take a bath within 6 hours.

Final treatment

1. Patient

After the treatment, the oil on the back of the patient should be wiped off. Ask the patient to avoid exposing to the cold, drink more warm boiled water, and refrain from strenuous exercise that day. After the patient has put on clothes, he or she should be led to the hall, rest for 5-10 minutes and drink a cup of warm boiled water or health-preserving herbal tea.

2. Arrangement of the flexible operating table and items

Clean the flexible operating table and place it in the specified location of the treatment room.

Arrange the suspended moxibustion device in time, check the burning of moxa sticks, and pay attention to fire prevention.

Tidy the room and bed unit.

Emergency plan

1. Allergy to essential oil

Stop using all essential oils immediately. For mild allergies, scrub the affected area with warm water; for severe allergies, give anti-allergic treatment.

2. Blisters due to moxibustion

Refer to the first section of this chapter "Spinal Regulation" for the management of blistering due to cupping.

Knowledge reserve (knowledge related to the procedure)

Level-1 knowledge reserve

The understanding of the holistic concept of Chinese Medicine and the importance of regulation of the back.

The running route of the governor vessel, location of key acupoints and indications.

The location and indications of Jiaji (EX-B2).

The running route of the bladder meridian, the location and function of Back-Shu acupoints.

Location, meridian tropism and indications of Fengchi (GB 20), Fengfu (DU 16), Jianjing (GB 21) and Tianzong(SI 11).

The function of the belt vessel.

The origins of the naming, locations and indications of Shenshu (BL 23) and

Mingmen (DU 4) and their importance in overall regulation.

The function of umbilical therapy.

Physiological functions of the five zang-organs.

Appendix of essential oil formula:

Liver. Add rosemary and bergamot essential oils to the jojoba essential oil.

Heart. Add neroli essential oil to jojoba essential oil.

Spleen. Add neroli and peppermint essential oils to jojoba oil.

Lung. Add tea tree and eucalyptus essential oils to jojoba oil.

Kidney. Add fennel essential oil to jojoba oil.

Evaluation standards of the techniques for the operation of five-element suspended moxibustion

See the table below of the evaluation standards of the techniques for the operation of five-element suspended moxibustion.

Evaluation standards of the techniques for the operation of five-element suspended moxibustion

Total score of the project (100 points)	Requirements	Score	Evaluation description	Deduction
Quality requirements (5 points)	Presentable appearance, elegant manner, amiable attitude, neat clothes, hand washing, mask wearing.	5	Points will be deducted as appropriate according to the completion condition.	

Continued

Total score of the project (100 points)		Requirements	Score	Evaluation description	Deduction
Pre-operation preparation (25 points)	Notification	Time required for treatment, effects, techniques, possible local symptoms, obtaining of patient's cooperation.	4	Points will be deducted as appropriate according to condition of notification.	
	Evaluation	(Four diagnostic methods) present history, past history, family history, history of allergies, pregnancy or menstrual period; skin condition of the operation region, tolerance to pain, etc.	10	Points will be deducted as appropriate according to the evaluation condition.	
	Items	1 flexible operating table. The upper layer: 1 treatment tray, 1 bottle of five-element suspended moxibustion essential oil, 2 smokeless moxa sticks, 1 alcohol lamp, 1 lighter, 1 umbilical powder, 1 special umbilical paste, 1 suspended moxibustion device The lower layer: 1 bed sheet, 2 towels (30 cm×70 cm), 1 bath towel and health-preserving clothes.	5	Points will be deducted as appropriate according to the condition of imperfect item preparation.	

Total score of the project (100 points)		Requirements	Score	Evaluation description	Deduction
Pre-operation preparation (25 points)	Patients and environment	Ask the patient about preparations before treatment, take a reasonable position, and loosen clothes. Keep the room tidy, protect privacy, keep warm and avoid convection wind.	6	3 points for each of the two items. Points will be deducted as appropriate if the answer is not perfect.	
Process of the operation (40 points)	Check the doctor's advice	Check the name and diagnosis, etc.	3	3 points will be deducted if check is not performed; points will be deducted as appropriate for incomplete contents.	
	Operation	Operate in accordance with the standard technical operating procedures (steps are attached, write the scores in detail).	25	Score according to the detailed points after the table.	

Continued

Total score of the project (100 points)		Requirements	Score	Evaluation description	Deduction
Process of the operation (40 points)	Observation	During the treatment, ask the patient about his or her feelings; comfort level and condition of pain;observe the skin condition of the operation region.	7	7 points will be deducted for failure to communicate with the patient, and points will be deducted as appropriate for incomplete contents.	
	After treatment	Ask the patient about his or her feelings and inform relevant precautions; assist the patient to take a comfortable position.	5	3 points will be deducted for failure to inform, and 2 points will be deducted for failure to arrange the patient's position.	
Post-operation (20 points)	Arrangement	Make up the bed unit, arrange things, clean and disinfect the items and put them in the original places, wash hands.	5	Points will be deducted as appropriate if the arrangement is not complete.	

Total score of the project (100 points)		Requirements	Score	Evaluation description	Deduction
Post-operation (20 points)	Evaluation	The operation part is accurate, the manipulation is skillful, the communication with the patient is good, and the patient feels that the expected goal is achieved.	5	Points will be deducted as appropriate if the evaluation is not complete.	
	Medical record	Detailed medical records to record treatment conditions, signature.	2	2 points will be deducted for failure to record; 1 point will be deducted for incomplete records.	
	Post-operation disposal	Used materials are handled in accordance with "Technical Standards for Disinfection of Medical Institutions".	8	For incorrect disposal method, 2 points will be deducted for each item.	
Theoretical questions (10 points)		Relevant knowledge of suspended moxibustion. Operation precautions of suspended moxibustion.	10	2 points will be deducted for incomplete answer of each question; 5 points will be deducted for no answer to each question.	

Total score:

Signature of the examiner: Assessment date:

Appendix with operation steps and scoring points:

1. Dredging of the meridians on the back

Step 1: Spread oil. (1 point)

Step 2: To dredge the governor vessel to the region of Baliao acupoints. (1.5 points)

Step 3: Push Jiaji (EX-B2) with the thumbs. (1.5 points)

Step 4: Push the bladder meridians with the thumbs. (1.5 points)

Step 5: Half clench the fists to dredge the bladder meridians. (1.5 points)

Step 6: Knead and press Jianjing (GB 21) and Tianzong(SI 11), dredge the medial line of the scapula. (2 points)

Step 7: Soothe the waist, press the acupoints at the waist and push the waist separately. (2 points)

Step 8: Rub heat Mingmen (DU 4). (1 point)

2. Dredging of the meridians on the abdomen

Step 1: Spread oil. (1 point)

Step 2: Push the conception vessel and stomach meridian. (2 points)

Step 3: Pressing the acupoints. (2 points)

Step 4: Knead the abdomen with the roots of the palms. (2 points)

Step 5: Pull and wipe the belt vessel. (2 points)

3. Abdominal moxibustion

Step 1: Drug administration on the umbilical region. (2 points)

Step 2: Ignite the smokeless moxa stick. (1 point)

Step 3: Connect the power supply to turn on the governor. (1 point)

Section 6 Five-Body Dredging

Name of the project

"Five-body" refers to the head, upper limbs and lower limbs, and also refer to tendons, vessels, muscles, skin, and bones. The five-body dredging is based on the "holistic concept" of Chinese Medicine and the characteristics of the running routes of the meridians to focus on the functions of the meridians and acupoints on the head, upper limbs, and lower limbs for the regulation of the body, which is a systematic regulation method by integrating dredging therapy of the meridians on the head, dredging of the meridians below the elbows and knees of the four limbs and foot reflexotherapy.

The function of the project

It has the function of dredging the meridians and collaterals, harmonizing qi and blood, balancing yin and yang, preventing diseases and preserve health.

Indications

It is applicable for dizziness, insomnia, fatigue, gastrointestinal dysfunction, cold hands and feet, headache and other sub-health conditions.

Standard technical operation procedures

1. Preparations

1.1 Pre-operation preparation of the operator

The operator should have good personal hygiene (including nail cutting), disinfect both hands, keep neat clothing and wear mask.

1.2 Items preparation

1 flexible operating table. ① The upper layer. 1 bucket of Chinese Medicine foot bath solution with water depth of 20-25 cm, 1 bottle of Collateral-Dredging Oil (10-30 ml), 1 scraping board for the head. ② The lower layer. 1 bed sheet, 4 towels (45 cm × 75 cm), 1 bath towel and health-preserving clothes.

1.3 Preparation for the patient

Instruct the patient to put on health-preserving clothes, loosen the hair, remove accessories and put away. Take a seat on the treatment bed, test the water temperature with both feet and take a foot bath.

2. Operation

Operate each technique for 3 times if there is no special instructions.

2.1 Operation on the head (15 minutes)

Massage on the head (8 minutes, 1 minute for each step)

Step 1: Press Yintang (EX-HN 3), pull and wipe Yintang (EX-HN 3) to Shenting (DU 24). Press Yintang (EX-HN 3) with the middle fingers of both hands, and then alternately pull and wipe Yintang (EX-HN 3) upward to Shenting (DU 24) by the middle fingers and ring fingers of both hands.

Step 2: Wipe the eyebrows to the Taiyang (EX-HN 5) and press Taiyang (EX-HN 5), Jingming (BL 1), Cuanzhu (BL 2), Yuyao (EX-HN 4), Sizhukong (SJ 23), pull and wipe the forehead. Separate the thumbs from the other four fingers of both hands, with the tips of the thumbs pointing down and the radial side of the thumb close to the forehead, wipe the eyebrows from the middle to the lateral and to Taiyang (EX-HN 5), press Taiyang (EX-HN 5) with the middle finger, press Jingming (BL 1), Cuanzhu (BL 2), Yuyao (EX-HN 4) and Sizhukong (SJ 23). The radial side of the thumbs pull and wipe the forehead from the middle to the lateral side of the forehead.

Step 3: Press the governor vessel and the bladder meridian, press and knead the forehead with the pulps of four fingers, press and knead tempus to the superior angle of the ear with digital joints. Press the governor vessel from Shenting (DU 24) to Baihui (GV 20) on the head with both thumbs, press the acupoints on the bladder meridian from Qucha (BL 4) to Luoque (BL 8); press and knead the tempus to the superior angle of the ear with the joints of four fingers of both hands.

Step 4: Sweep the gallbladder meridian with the hand and press Shuaigu (GB 8). Bend the four fingers naturally, sweep the gallbladder meridian on one side of the head with the pulps of the fingers, operate the same on the right gallbladder meridian, point-press Shuaigu (GB 8) with the middle finger.

Step 5: Press Tinggong (SI 19) and Tinghui (GB 2), rub and knead the ears and press

Yifeng (SJ 17). Press Tinggong (SI 19) and Tinghui (GB 2) with the middle fingers of both hands, pinch the roots of the ears to quickly rub the ears up and down until they become hot with the index and middle fingers of both hands, and then press Yifeng (SJ 17) with the middle fingers.

Step 6: Grasp and knead the nape to Dazhui (DU 14), press Fengchi (GB 20) and Fengfu (DU 16). Place one hand on the top of the head to fix the head. The thumb of the other hand is arched with the other four fingers. Grasp and knead the nape muscles to Dazhui (DU 14), press Fengchi (GB 20) and Fengfu (DU 16) with the thumb.

Step 7: Grasp and knead the trapezius to the upper arm. Grasp and knead trapezius to the upper arms with the junction parts between the thumbs and index fingers of both hands.

Step 8: Knock on the head to end. Stand the palms to face each other with fingertips facing forward, knock on the head rhythmically with the ulnar borders of the metacarpophalangeal joints of little fingers.

Scraping on the head (7 minutes)

Step 1: Press Baihui (GV 20), scrap from Baihui (GV 20) forward to Shenting (DU 24). Fix the head with one hand and hold the scraping board in the other. Use the corner of the scraping board as the focus point to press Baihui (GV 20), and then scrape from Baihui (GV 20) to Shenting (DU 24) of the anterior hairline. (1 minute)

Step 2: Scrape the head radially from Baihui (GV 20). Scrape the head radially from Baihui (GV 20) clockwise with a scraping board. (2 minutes)

Step 3: Scrape the forehead. Scrape the area 1 cm anterior and posterior to the anterior hairline with one corner of the scraping board, from the left Touwei (ST 8) to the right Touwei (ST 8) gradually and to and fro. (1 minute)

Step 4: Scrape the governor vessel, the bladder meridian and the gallbladder meridian. Scrape the left meridians first and then the right. The scraping board scrapes along the running routes of the governor vessel, the bladder meridian and the gallbladder meridian, from the anterior hairline to the posterior hairline and from the left to the right. (2 minutes)

Step 5: Comb the hair to finish the procedure. Use the teeth part of the scraping board to comb the patient's hair neatly. (1 minute)

2.2 Operation on the upper limbs (mainly operate the part below the elbows and knees, left first and then right) (20 minutes)

Step 1: Press and knead the lung meridian with the thumbs, press Chize (LU 5) and Taiyuan (LU 9). Knead the lung meridian with the thumb from Chize (LU 5) to Taiyuan (LU 9) and press these two acupoints with the thumb.

Step 2: Press and knead the large intestine meridian, and digital-press Yangxi (LI 5) and Quchi (LI 11). Knead the large intestine meridian with the thumb from Yangxi (LI 5) to Quchi (LI 11), and press Yangchi (SJ 4) and Quchi (LI 11) with the thumb.

Step 3: Press and knead the pericardium meridian, and digital-press Quze (PC 3) and Neiguan (PC 6). Knead the pericardium meridian with the thumb from Quze (PC 3) to Neiguan (PC 6), and then press these two acupoints.

Step 4: Knead the triple energizer meridian with the thumb, press Waiguan (SJ 5) and Tianjing (SJ 10). Knead the triple energizer meridian with the thumb from Waiguan (SJ 5) to Tianjing (SJ 10), and press these two acupoints.

Step 5: Knead the heart meridian with the thumb and press Shaohai (HT 3) and Shenmen (HT 7). Knead the heart meridian with the thumb from Shaohai (HT 3) to Shenmen (HT 7), and press these acupoints with the thumb.

Step 6: Knead the small intestine meridian with the thumb, digital-press Yanggu (SI 5) and Xiaohai (SI 8). Knead the small intestine meridian with the thumb from Yanggu (SI 5) to Xiaohai (SI 8), and press these acupoints with the thumb.

Step 7: Knead the forearm with the palm, press the Yaotongdian (EX-UE 7), Laozhen (EX-UE 8) and Hegu (LI 4).

Step 8: Push the palm, and push the five fingers separately with the thumb, rub and knead the root of the palm; press Laogong (PC 8), knock the palm, tract the wrist. Push the center of the palm and push the five fingers separately with the thumb; fix the patient's wrist with one hand and cross the patient's five fingers with the other hand, rub the root of the patient's palm with the doctor's palm root, press Laogong (PC 8), knock the patient's palm with the doctor's palm, tract the patient's wrist.

Step 9: Rub and knead the fingers and tract the interphalangeal joints. Rub and knead the patient's fingers with the doctor's thumb and index finger from the patient's thumb to the little finger, and then tract the interphalangeal joints.

Step 10: Perform kneading, patting, shaking, and traction on the upper limbs to end the procedure.

After the foot bath is over, dry the feet with a towel and start the operation on the lower limbs.

2.3 Operation on the lower limbs (5 minutes)

Step 1: Knead the patella with the five fingers of both hands. Fix the patella with the five fingers of both hands, and knead the patella in a circular motion.

Step 2: Knead Xiyan (EX-LE 5). Use the thumbs and index fingers of both hands to knead the medial and lateral Xiyan (EX-LE 5) acupoints.

Step 3: Knead Zusanli (ST 36) and Sanyinjiao (SP 6). Knead Zusanli (ST 36) and Sanyinjiao (SP 6) on both sides with the thumbs of both hands.

Step 4: Grasp and knead the calves with both hands. Grasp and knead the medial and lateral Xiyan (EX-LE 5) acupoints with both hands to Jiexi (ST 41).

Step 5: Move the ankle joints. Hold the ends of both feet, and make the feet turn left, turn right, dorsiflex and plantarflex.

Step 6: Knock the lateral side of the calves with empty fists. Knock the lateral side of the calves with both hands.

2.4 Operation on the foot, the operation sequence is the sole of the foot, the medial side of the foot, the lateral side of the foot, the dorsum of the foot (left foot first and then right foot), for 40 minutes and 20 minutes for each foot

Soles of the foot

Press the center of the left foot to detect the patient's heart condition, and determine the comfortable force for the patient.

Step 1: Press the Adrenal Gland acupoint. The Adrenal Gland is point-like acupoint. Clench the right fist and adduct the thumb, press with the second interphalangeal joint of the index finger.

Step 2: Scrape Coeliac Plexus acupoint. The Coeliac Plexus is a face-like acupoint. Clench the right fist and adduct the thumb, scrape the left and right semicircular arcs with the second interphalangeal joint of the index finger.

Step 3: Press the Kidney acupoint. The Kidney acupoint is point-like acupoint. Clench the right fist and adduct the thumb, press with the second interphalangeal joint of the index finger.

Step 4: Wipe the Ureter acupoint. The Ureter acupoint is a linear acupoint. Clench the right fist and adduct the thumb, use the second interphalangeal joint of the index finger to scrape from the kidney to the bladder in an arc.

Step 5: Press the Bladder acupoint. The Bladder acupoint is point-like. Clench the right fist and adduct the thumb, press with the second interphalangeal joint of the index finger.

Step 6: Push the Urethra and Perineum acupoints. The Urethra and Perineum acupoints are linear. Push upward in an arc with the pulp of the right thumb from the bladder reflex area.

Step 7: Scrape the Forehead (Frontal Sinus) acupoint. The Forehead (Frontal Sinus) acupoint is point-shaped. The left thumb and the other four fingers are fixed on the toes of the left foot, and the right hand clenches to an empty fist to scrape horizontally with the interphalangeal joint of the thumb.

Step 8: Push the Trigeminus acupoint. The Trigeminus acupoint is linear. Push straightly down from the toe-end with the right thumb.

Step 9: Digital-press the Cerebellum and Brainstem acupoints. The Cerebellum and Brainstem acupoint are point-like. Clench the right fist and adduct the thumb, digital-press with the second interphalangeal joint of the index finger.

Step 10: Push the Neck acupoint. The Neck acupoint is linear. One-way horizontal push is performed medially with the pulp of the right thumb.

Step 11: Push the Nose acupoint. The Nose acupoint is linear. Push it along the edge of the nail of the right thumb.

Step 12: Digital-press the Brain acupoint. The Brain acupoint is point-like. Clench the right fist and adduct the thumb, digital-press with the second interphalangeal joint of the index finger.

Step 13: Digital-press Hypophysis Cerebri acupoint. The Hypophysis Cerebri acupoint is point-like. Clench the right fist and adduct the thumb, digital-press with the second interphalangeal joint of the index finger.

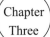

Step 14: Scrape the Esophagus and Trachea acupoints. The Esophagus and Trachea acupoints are linear. Clench the right hand into an empty fist and adduct the thumb, perform one-way scraping with the second interphalangeal joint of the index finger.

Step 15: Scrape the Parathyroid Gland acupoint. The Parathyroid Gland acupoint is linear. Clench the right hand into an empty fist and adduct the thumb, perform one-way scraping with the second interphalangeal joint of the index finger.

Step 16: Scrape the Thyroid Gland acupoint. The Thyroid Gland acupoint is linear. Clench the right hand into an empty fist and adduct the thumb, perform one-way scraping with the second interphalangeal joint of the index finger.

Step 17: Scrape the Head acupoint. The Head acupoint is point-like. The left thumb and the other four fingers are fixed on the toes of the left foot. Clench the right hand into an empty fist, scrape transversely with the interphalangeal joint of the thumb.

Step 18: Digital-press the Eye acupoint. The Eye acupoint is point-like. Clench the right fist and adduct the thumb, press with the second interphalangeal joint of the index finger.

Step 19: Digital-press the Ear acupoint. The Ear acupoint is point-like. Clench the right fist and adduct the thumb, digital-press with the second interphalangeal joint of the index finger.

Step 20: Scrape the Trapezius acupoint. The Trapezius acupoint is linear. Clench the right hand into an empty fist and adduct the thumb. Perform one-way scraping from the lateral to the medial with the first and second interphalangeal joints of the index finger.

Step 21: Push the Lung and Bronchi acupoints. The Lung and Bronchi acupoints are shaped like the Chinese character " 人 ". With the left and right thumbs facing each other, push and squeeze from both sides of the pelma to the middle region, then turn around the thumbs and push straightly up to the root of toes.

Step 22: Digital-press the Heart (Right Liver) acupoint. The Heart acupoint is point-like. Clench the right hand into an empty fist and adduct the thumb, digital-press with the second interphalangeal joint of the index finger.

Step 23: Digital-press the Spleen (Right Gallbladder) acupoint. The Spleen acupoint is point-like. Clench the right hand into an empty fist and adduct the thumb, digital-press with the second interphalangeal joint of the index finger.

Step 24: Scrape the Stomach acupoint. The Stomach acupoint is face-like. Clench the right hand into an empty fist and adduct the thumb, perform one-way straight downward scraping with the second interphalangeal joint of the index finger.

Step 25: Scrape the Pancreas acupoint. The Pancreas acupoint is face-like. Clench the right hand into an empty fist and adduct the thumb, perform one-way straight downward scraping with the second interphalangeal joint of the index finger.

Step 26: Scrape the Duodenum acupoint. The Duodenum acupoint is face-like. Clench the right hand into an empty fist and adduct the thumb, perform one-way straight downward scraping with the second interphalangeal joint of the index finger.

Step 27: Scrape the Small Intestine acupoint. The Small Intestine acupoint is face-shaped. The left hand performs to fix, the right hand clenches into a fist and the thumb is adducted, the second interphalangeal joints of the remaining four fingers perform one-way straight downward scraping.

Step 28: Scrape the Transverse Colon (Right Ascending Colon) acupoint. The Transverse Colon acupoint is linear. The interphalangeal joint of the right index finger performs one-way horizontal scraping to the lateral side of the pelma.

Step 29: Scrape the Descending Colon (Right Transverse Colon) acupoint. The Descending Colon acupoint is linear. The interphalangeal joint of the right index finger performs one-way vertical scraping to the lateral and superior border of the heel.

Step 30: Scrape the Sigmoid Colon acupoint. the Sigmoid Colon acupoint is linear. The interphalangeal joint of the right index finger performs one-way vertical scraping to the medial side of the heel.

Step 31: Digital-press Insomnia acupoint. The Insomnia acupoint is point-like. Clench the right hand into an empty fist and adduct the thumb, digital-press with the second interphalangeal joint of the index finger.

Step 32: Digital-press the Reproduction acupoint. The Reproduction acupoint is point-like. Clench the right hand into an empty fist and adduct the thumb, digital-press with the second interphalangeal joint of the index finger.

The medial side of the foot

Step 1: Push the Cervical Spine acupoint. This acupoint is linear. Perform one-way straight pushing on the medial side from front to back with the pulp of the right thumb.

Step 2: Push the Thoracic Spine acupoint. This acupoint is linear. Perform one-way straight pushing on the medial side from front to back with the pulp of the right thumb.

Step 3: Push the Lumbar Spine acupoint. This acupoint is linear. Perform one-way straight pushing on the medial side from front to back with the pulp of the right thumb.

Step 4: Push the Sacrum acupoint. This acupoint is linear. Perform one-way straight pushing on the medial side from front to back with the pulp of the right thumb.

Step 5: Knead and press the Uterus (Prostate) acupoint. This acupoint is face-like. Knead and press with the pulp of the right thumb in a circular motion.

Step 6: Push the Medial Rectum and Anus acupoints. The Medial Rectum and Anus acupoints area linear. Perform one-way straight pushing from the medial side of the ankle to the medial side of the calf with the pulp of the right thumb.

The lateral side of the foot

Step 1: Push the Shoulder acupoint. The Shoulder acupoint is linear. Perform one-way straight pushing from the upper to the lower with the second interphalangeal joint of the right index finger.

Step 2: Digital-press the Elbow acupoint. The Elbow acupoint is linear. Digital-press the inferior of the shoulder and superior of the knee with the second interphalangeal joints of the index finger and middle finger.

Step 3: Scrape the Knee Joint acupoint. The Knee Joint acupoint is linear. Scrape in an arc from the upper to the bottom with the second interphalangeal joint surface of the right index finger.

Step 4: Press and knead the Ovary (Testicle) acupoint. The Ovary (Testicle) acupoint is face-shaped. Knead and press in a annular motion with the pulp of the thumb.

Step 5: Push the Scaplula acupoint. The Scapula acupoint is linear. Perform one-way straight pushing from the lower to the upper with both thumbs in parallel up and down.

Step 6: Push the Lower Abdomen acupoint. The Lower Abdomen acupoint is linear. Perform one-way straight pushing from the lateral side of the ankle upward to the lateral side of the calf with the pulp of the right thumb.

Dorsum of the foot

Step 1: Push the Upper Palate and Lower Palate acupoints. Keep the two thumbs in parallel, fingertips of both hands facing each other and the pulps of the fingers of both hands opposite to each other, and then push horizontally.

Step 2: Digital-press the Tonsil acupoint. Digital-press the acupoint with the pulps of both thumbs.

Step 3: Digital-press the Throat acupoint. Digital-press the acupoint with the pulps of both thumbs.

Step 4: Knead and press the Chest and Breast acupoints. Knead and press in a annular motion with the pulps of both thumbs.

Step 5: Push the Diaphragm acupoint. Push separately from the medial to the lateral with the radial borders of the second interphalangeal joints of both index fingers.

Step 6: Digital-press Jiexi (ST 41) with the thumb.

Standards of working language

1. Before treatment

Hello, sir (madam)! I'm your regulation physician. I'm very happy to be at your service. What we are doing today is the project of five-body dredging. The project of five-body dredging is to apply techniques combined with reflex zone therapy to dredge the meridians of the head, upper limbs, and lower limbs to balance yin and yang, harmonize qi and blood, promote blood circulation and dredge collaterals, prevent disease and preserve health. It has a good relaxing effect on insomnia and headaches caused by long-term over-thinking, stress, and staying up late.

The treatment duration is about 80 minutes. Do you need to go to the bathroom? (No.)

Sir (madam), let's start. Please change into health-preserving clothes. I will help you store your valuables. After putting on health-preserving clothes, lean back on the sofa.

2. Treatment

Follow the steps in the treatment combined with language art.

Do you feel uncomfortable in any way? I can give you regulation based on syndrome differentiation according to your condition.

2.1 Massage and scraping on the head

What I'm doing for you now is pressing Baihui (GV 20). The head is the convergence of all yang and communication of various meridians, which plays an important role in controlling and regulating the life activities of the human body. Massage and scraping the meridians and acupoints on the head can promote rising of clear yang, harmonizing various meridians, clearing the mind and enhancing memory. Do you think the force is OK?

2.2 Massage the upper limbs and lower limbs

Massage on the upper limbs is mainly to dredge the three yin and three yang meridians of the hands. There are many acupoints on each meridian. For example, the acupoint pressed now is Chize (LU 5) which is a acupoint of the lung meridian and can regulate the function of the lung. Neiguan (PC 6) on the pericardium meridian can regulate the function of the heart. By dredging the meridians and pressing key acupoints, it can improve qi and blood circulation of the limbs and achieve the purpose of disease prevention and health care. Massage on the lower limbs is mainly to dredge the three yin and three yang meridians of the feet. Among them, Zusanli (ST 36) of the stomach meridian of foot Yangming has the function of strengthening the spleen and stomach, strengthening the body and harmonizing qi and blood. Sanyinjiao (SP 6) on the spleen meridian of foot Taiyin is a commonly-used acupoint in gynecology and plays an important role in the disease regulation and health care for the females.

2.3 Massage on the foot reflex zone

According to Chinese Medicine, the three yin meridians and three yang meridians of the feet start and end at the feet respectively, which maintains the circulation of qi and blood in human body through the relationship among the meridians and collaterals. The diseases of the viscera can influence each other through the meridians. Dredging the meridians and regulating qi and blood can achieve the effect of treating the diseases of the viscera.

3. Concluding remarks

Sir (madam), the project of five-body dredging has been completed. How do you feel? Thanks for your cooperation. If you have any comments and suggestions, please let us know and we will improve actively.

Cautions

Before the treatment, pay attention to whether the room lighting and temperature are appropriate.

Pay attention to rest. Do not stay up late, keep your mood happy, keep warm and avoid wind and coldness.

Keep your mood happy, work and rest on time, and do not wash hair or take a bath within 6 hours after treatment.

Final treatment

1. Patient

At the end of the treatment, the Collateral-Dredging Oil on the patient's feet should be wiped clean. Ask the patient to avoid exposing to cold, drink more warm boiled water, and refrain from strenuous exercise that day. After the patient has put on his clothes, he or she should be led to the hall, rest for 5-10 minutes and drink a cup of warm boiled water or health-preserving herbal tea.

2. Arrangement of the flexible operating table and items

Clean the flexible operating table and place it in the specified location of the treatment room.

After cleaning the scraping board, scrub it with alcohol for disinfection, and dry it for later use.

Tidy the room and bed unit.

Emergency plan

1. Allergy to collateral-dredging oil

Refer to the treatment method in the first section of this chapter "Tuina of the meridian sinews".

Knowledge reserve (knowledge related to the procedure)

Level-1 knowledge reserve

The holistic concept of the five bodies and its importance.

The running routes of the twelve meridians especially the regions on the head and below the elbows and knees of the four limbs, the locations of the acupoints and indications.

Specific location of the foot reflection area.

Evaluation standards of the techniques for the operation of five-body dredging

See the table below for the evaluation standards of the techniques for the operation of five-body dredging.

Evaluation standards of the techniques for the operation of five-body dredging

Total score of the project (100 points)	Requirements	Score	Evaluation description	Deduction
Quality requirements (5 points)	Presentable appearance, elegant manner, amiable attitude, neat clothes, hand washing, mask wearing.	5	Points will be deducted as appropriate according to the completion condition.	

Continued

Total score of the project (100 points)		Requirements	Score	Evaluation description	Deduction
Pre-operation preparation (25 points)	Notification	Time required for treatment, effects, techniques, possible local symptoms, obtaining of patient's cooperation.	4	Points will be deducted as appropriate according to condition of notification.	
	Evaluation	(Four diagnostic methods) present history, past history, family history, history of allergies, pregnancy or menstrual period; skin condition of the operation region, tolerance to pain, etc.	10	be deducted as appropriate according to the evaluation condition.	
	Items	1 flexible operating table. The upper layer: 1 bucket of Chinese medicine foot bath water, with depth of 20-25 cm, a bottle of Collateral-Dredging Oil(10-30 ml), and 1 scalp scraping board. The lower layer: 1 bed sheet, 3 towels (30 cm×70 cm), 1 bath towel and health-preserving clothes.	5	Points will be deducted as appropriate according to the condition of imperfect item preparation.	

Total score of the project (100 points)		Requirements	Score	Evaluation description	Deduction
Pre-operation preparation (25 points)	Patients and environment	Ask the patient about preparations before treatment, take a reasonable position, and loosen clothes. Keep the room tidy, protect privacy, keep warm and avoid convection wind.	6	3 points for each of the two items. Points will be deducted as appropriate if the answer is not perfect.	
Process of the operation (40 points)	Check the doctor's advice	Check the name and diagnosis, etc.	3	3 points will be deducted if check is not performed; points will be deducted as appropriate for incomplete contents.	
	Operation	Operate in accordance with the standard technical operating procedures (steps are attached, write the scores in detail).	25	Score according to the detailed points after the table.	

Continued

Total score of the project (100 points)		Requirements	Score	Evaluation description	Deduction
Process of the operation (40 points)	Observation	During the treatment, ask the patient about his or her feelings; comfort level and condition of pain;observe the skin condition of the operation region.	7	7 points will be deducted for failure to communicate with the patient, and points will be deducted as appropriate for incomplete contents.	
	After treatment	Ask the patient about his or her feelings and inform relevant precautions; assist the patient to take a comfortable position.	5	3 points will be deducted for failure to inform, and 2 points will be deducted for failure to arrange the patient's position.	
Post-operation (20 points)	Arrangement	Make up the bed unit, arrange things, clean and disinfect the items and put them in the original places, wash hands.	5	Points will be deducted as appropriate if the arrangement is not complete.	

Total score of the project (100 points)		Requirements	Score	Evaluation description	Deduction
Post-operation (20 points)	Evaluation	The operation part is accurate, the manipulation is skillful, the communication with the patient is good, and the patient feels that the expected goal is achieved.	5	Points will be deducted as appropriate if the evaluation is not complete.	
	Medical record	Detailed medical records to record treatment conditions, signature.	2	2 points will be deducted for failure to record; 1 point will be deducted for incomplete records.	
	Post-operation disposal	Used materials are handled in accordance with "Technical Standards for Disinfection of Medical Institutions".	8	For incorrect disposal method, 2 points will be deducted for each item.	
Theoretical questions (10 points)		Relevant knowledge of five-body dredging.\n\nOperation precautions for the five-body dredging.	10	2 points will be deducted for incomplete answer of each question; 5 points will be deducted for no answer to each question.	

Total score:

Signature of the examiner: Assessment date:

Appendix with operation steps and scoring points:

1. Operation on the head

Massage on the head (4 points)

Step 1: Press Yintang (EX-HN 3), pull and wipe Yintang (EX-HN 3) to Shenting (DU 24).

Step 2: Wipe the eyebrows to the Taiyang (EX-HN 5) and press Taiyang (EX-HN 5), press Jingming (BL 1), Cuanzhu (BL 2), Yuyao (EX-HN 4), Sizhukong (SJ 23), pull and wipe the forehead.

Step 3: Press the governor vessel and the bladder meridian, press and knead the tempus with the pulps of four fingers, press and knead tempus to the superior angle of the ear with digital joints.

Step 4: Sweep the gallbladder meridian with the hand and press Shuaigu (GB 8).

Step 5: Press Tinggong (SI 19) and Tinghui (GB 2), rub and knead the ears and press Yifeng (SJ 17).

Step 6: Grasp and knead the nape to Dazhui (DU 14), press Fengchi (GB 20) and Fengfu (DU 16).

Step 7: Grasp and knead the trapezius to the upper arm. Grasp and knead trapezius to the upper arms with the junction parts between the thumbs and index fingers of both hands.

Step 8: Knock on the head to finish.

Scraping on the head (3 points)

Step 1: Press Baihui (GV 20), scrap from Baihui (GV 20) forward to Shenting (DU 24).

Step 2: Scrape the head radially from Baihui (GV 20).

Step 3: Scrape the forehead.

Step 4: Scrape the governor vessel, the bladder meridian and the gallbladder meridian. Scrape the left meridians first and then the right.

Step 5: Comb the hair to finish the procedure.

2. Operations on the upper limbs (5 points)

Step 1: Press and knead the lung meridian with the thumb, digital-press Chize (LU 5) and Taiyuan (LU 9).

Step 2: Press and knead the large intestine meridian, and digital-press Yangxi (LI 5) and Quchi (LI 11).

Step 3: Press and knead the pericardium meridian, and digital-press Quze (PC 3) and Neiguan (PC 6).

Step 4: Knead the triple energizer meridian with the thumb, digital-press Waiguan (SJ 5) and Tianjing (SJ 10).

Step 5: Knead the heart meridian with the thumb and digital-press Shaohai (HT 3) and Shenmen (HT 7).

Step 6: Knead the small intestine meridian with the thumb, digital-press Yanggu (SI 5) and Xiaohai (SI 8).

Step 7: Knead the forearm with the palm, press the Yaotongdian (EX-UE 7), Laozhen (EX-UE 8) and Hegu (LI 4).

Step 8: Push the palm, and push the five fingers separately with the thumb, rub and knead the root of the palm; press Laogong (PC 8), knock the palm, tract the wrist.

Step 9: Rub and knead the fingers and tract the interphalangeal joints.

Step 10: Operate kneading, patting, shaking, and traction on the upper limbs to end the procedure.

3. Operation on the lower limbs (3 points)

Step 1: Knead the patella with the five fingers of both hands.

Step 2: Knead Xiyan (EX-LE 5).

Step 3: Knead Zusanli (ST 36) and Sanyinjiao (SP 6).

Step 4: Grasp and knead the calves with both hands.

Step 5: Move the ankle joints.

Step 6: Knock the lateral side of the calves with empty fists.

4. Operation on the foot: The operation sequence is the sole of the foot, the medial side of the foot, the lateral side of the foot and the dorsum of the foot (first left and then right, a total of 10 points, 5 points for each side)

Soles of the foot

Step 1: Press the Adrenal Gland acupoint.

Step 2: Scrape Coeliac Plexus acupoint.

Step 3: Press the Kidney acupoint.

Step 4: Wipe the Ureter acupoint.

Step 5: Press the Bladder acupoint.

Step 6: Push the Urethra and Perineum acupoints.

Step 7: Scrape the Forehead (Frontal Sinus) acupoint.

Step 8: Push the Trigeminus acupoint.

Step 9: Digital-press the Cerebellum and Brainstem acupoints.

Step 10: Push the Neck acupoint.

Step 11: Push the Nose acupoint.

Step 12: Digital-press the Brain acupoint.

Step 13: Digital-press Hypophysis Cerebri acupoint.

Step 14: Scrape the Esophagus and Trachea acupoints.

Step 15: Scrape the Parathyroid Gland acupoint.

Step 16: Scrape the Thyroid Gland acupoint.

Step 17: Scrape the Head acupoint.

Step 18: Digital-press the Eye acupoint.

Step 19: Digital-press the Ear acupoint.

Step 20: Scrape the Trapezius acupoint.

Step 21: Push the Lung and Bronchi acupoints.

Step 22: Digital-press the Heart (Right Liver) acupoint.

Step 23: Digital-press the Spleen (Right Gallbladder) acupoint.

Step 24: Scrape the Stomach acupoint.

Step 25: Scrape the Pancreas acupoint.

Step 26: Scrape the Duodenum acupoint.

Step 27: Scrape the Small Intestine acupoint.

Step 28: Scrape the Transverse Colon (Right Ascending Colon) acupoint.

Step 29: Scrape the Descending Colon (Right Transverse Colon) acupoint.

Step 30: Scrap the Sigmoid Colon acupoint (no right).

Step 31: Digital-press Insomnia acupoint.

Step 32: Digital-press the Reproduction acupoint.

The medial side of the foot

Step 1: Push the Cervical Spine acupoint.

Step 2: Push the Thoracic Spine acupoint.

Step 3: Push the Lumbar Spine acupoint.

Step 4: Push the Sacrum acupoint.

Step 5: Knead and press the Uterus (Prostate) acupoint.

Step 6: Push the medial Rectum and Anus acupoints.

The lateral side of the foot

Step 1: Push the Shoulder acupoint.

Step 2: Digital-press the Elbow acupoint.

Step 3: Scrape the Knee Joint acupoint.

Step 4: Press and knead the Ovary (Testicle) acupoint.

Step 5: Push the Scapula acupoint.

Step 6: Push the Lower Abdomen acupoint.

Dorsum of the foot

Step 1: Push the Upper Palate and Lower Palate acupoints.

Step 2: Digital-press the Tonsil acupoint.

Step 3: Digital-press the Throat acupoint.

Step 4: Knead and press the Chest and Breast acupoints.

Step 5: Push the Diaphragm acupoint.

Step 6: Digital-press Jiexi (ST 41) with the thumb.

Section 7 Regulation with Medicated Bath

Name of the project

Regulation with medicated bath is a kind of unique regulation of the meridians and collaterals of the whole body by means of the combination of traditional techniques of Chinese Medicine and traditional medicated bath, adding aromatherapy, musicotherapy and benign stimuli of vision, touch, smell and hearing.

The function of the project

It has the function of dredging the meridians, smoothing qi and blood, balancing the internal and external, coordinating the viscera and enhancing vitality.

Indications

It is suitable for poor immunity, cold body, insomnia, gastrointestinal dysfunction, anxiety, fatigue, etc.

Contraindications

Those with open injuries and local wounds that have not healed should not be given this treatment to prevent infection.

This therapy is not suitable for women during menstruation and pregnancy.

Patients with cardiovascular and cerebrovascular diseases such as hypertension and heart disease. Patients with cardiopulmonary insufficiency and weak constitution should not be given this treatment to prevent accidents.

It is not advisable for the elderly, the weak and children. For special cases requiring this treatment, the patient should be accompanied by family members, and the treatment duration should not be too long.

People who are allergic to Chinese medicine should be given this treatment with caution. Those who appear skin irritation during the treatment should be stopped the treatment and consult a physician in time.

This treatment should not be given within 30 minutes of an empty stomach or after a full meal, which can easily cause dizziness or fatigue.

Patients with high fever and profuse sweating should not be given this treatment to prevent collapse.

Standard technical operation procedures

1. Preparations

1.1 Pre-operation preparation for the operator

The operator should perform personal hygiene (including nail cutting), disinfect hands, wear neat clothes and a mask.

1.2 Items preparation

1 flexible operating table. ① The upper layer. 1 bottle of Collateral-Dredging Oil 10-30ml, 1 bottle of shower gel, 1 bottle of shampoo, 1 aroma lamp, 1 music player, 1 disposable medicated bath cover, 1 body mask, 1 bottle of body lotion. ② The lower level. 1 shower cap, 1 bed sheet, 2 bath towels, 1 quilt, 2 towels (30 cm × 70 cm), 2 disposable underwear, and health-preserving clothes.

1.3 Preparation of the patient

Ask the patient to change clothes, take a bath, mind the step to prevent slipping.

2. Operation

2.1 Bathing (40 minutes)

Step 1: Prepare bath water, turn on the music, incense lamp, and prepare tea.

Step 2: Put a disposable medicated bath cover in the bath tub, add appropriate amount of water (depending on the specific conditions of the patient, generally add water to 1/2-2/3 of the medicated bath tub), and put the medical solution (appropriate amount for adult formula, reduced for children, water temperature 37-40°C, 38°C is the best) (with prescriptions: Qi-Benefiting and Fatigue-Relieving Formula, Shoulder-Relaxing and Spasm-Relieving Formula, Uterus-Warming and Cold-Dissipating Formula, Liver-Soothing and Depression-Relieving Formula, Heart-Nourishing and Mind-Tranquilizing Formula, etc.).

Step 3: After adjusting the water temperature, instruct the patient to take a bath. Ask the patient about the bathing situation at any time. If there is any discomfort, stop bathing immediately and give corresponding treatment according to specific situation.

2.2 Massage on the back: Twice for each step (10 minutes)

Step 1: Spread oil and soothe the back area. ① The doctor stands beside the head of the bed, takes an appropriate amount of oil on the palms, rubs the palms together (the palms are fully spread with oil which won't drop and it should not drop on the patient's back, hair and sheets). Open two palms and put them on the bladder meridians besides the spine, fully stick to the back from Dazhui (DU 14) horizontally in sequence of roots of the palms, palms, fingers and fingertips, then leave the back by following the above order (the four fingertips won't leave the back except the fingertip of thumb), repeat in the above sequence to stick to the back, leave the back until the lumbosacral region, allowing the back region where both palms pass through are spread with oil. ② Raise both hands, put the fingertips of both palms opposite to each other and stick close to the back on both sides of the spine, push down horizontally from Dazhui (DU 14) to the lumbosacral region, turn palms to be parallel to the spine and pull back to the level of Dazhui (DU 14). Separate the palms to the shoulders and wrap the shoulders, lift to Fengchi (GB 20) by following the direction of the trapezius, and digital-press Fengchi (GB 20) with middle finger.

Step 2: Rub the governor vessel with hands overlapping to dredge the governor vessel. Place the thumbs of both hands adjacent on the governor vessel in the direction perpendicular to the spine, stick the fingertips of the remaining four fingers outwards on the back. The thumbs start from Dazhui (DU 14) and push evenly the governor vessel to the Baliao area of the lumbosacral region. Overlap the two hands with the left hand above and rub warm from Dazhui (DU 14) to Baliao area.

Step 3: Push the bladder meridian and pull back the hand to the fingertips to detoxify. Push or separately push the first line of the bladder meridian on both sides with both thumbs. The other four fingertips are attached outward to the back to the lumbosacral area, and the palms of the remaining four fingers except the thumbs are placed together and attached outward to the back on both sides, push along the arm to fingertips to detoxify.

Step 4: Dredge the hypochondriac regions. Use thumbs and index fingers to alternately push along the ribs of both sides of the body (under the armpit to the free edge of the 12 ribs).

Step 5: Press Dazhui (DU 14) and the acupoints on the first lateral line of the bladder meridian on the back with both thumbs.

Step 6: Push the back in Tai Chi style. Push the entire back with both hands alternately by drawing circles.

Step 7: Digital-press Mingmen (DU 4) with both thumbs.

2.3 Massage on the buttocks: Twice for each step (5 minutes)

Step 1: Spread oil. Spread the Collateral-Dredging Oil with both hands in fan shape.

Step 2: Digital-press the acupoints. Digital-press Huantiao (GB 30) and Chengfu (BL 36) with the thumb.

Step 3: Lift the buttocks. Push, knead and pull up the lateral side of the buttocks with both hands.

Step 4: Press Huantiao (GB 30) and Chengfu (BL 36) with both thumbs. Soothe the back to end the procedure.

2.4 Massage the posterior of the leg: Twice for each step (5 minutes)

Step 1: Spread oil. Spread the Collateral-Dredging Oil with both hands alternately in straight line.

Step 2: Digital-press Chengfu (BL 36), Weizhong (BL 40) and Chengshan (BL 57).

Step 3: Dredge the bladder meridians on the posterior part of the legs with both hands.

Step 4: Press Chengfu (BL 36), Weizhong (BL 40) and Chengshan (BL 57), grasp and knead the muscles of the calves.

2.5 Massage on the chest: Find the nodules carefully, twice for each step (5 minutes)

Step 1: Spread oil.

Step 2: Digital-press Tiantu (RN 22), Danzhong (RN 17), Rugen (ST 18), Wuyi (ST 15) and Yunmen (LU 2).

Step 3: Lift the breasts. Put the four fingers together, lift and pull with both hands alternately from the lateral to the medial.

Step 4: To find out nodules. Gently knead the breast with the pulps of four fingers. If there is nodule, instruct the patient for further examination.

Step 5: Digital-press Tiantu (RN 22), Danzhong (RN 17), Rugen (ST 18), Wuyi (ST 15) and Yunmen (LU 2).

2.6 Massage on the abdomen: Twice for each step (5 minutes)

Step 1: Spread oil.

Step 2: Digital-press Shangwan (RN 13), Zhongwan (RN 12), Xiawan (RN 10), Qihai (RN 6) and Guanyuan (RN 4).

Step 3: Dredge the conception vessel. Push the conception vessel from Shangwan (RN 13) downward to Zhongji (RN 3) with the roots of both palms.

Step 4: Dredge the side waist. Pull from the side of the waist along the upper edge of the highest point of the iliac bone to Zhongji (RN 3), then perform on the other side.

Step 5: Push and knead the side waist with both hands.

Step 6: Rub warm Shenque (RN 8) with both hands.

Step 7: To expel toxin. Push separately to the side waist with the roots of both palms, and then pull back from the waist to remove toxin.

2.7 Massage on the arms: Twice for each step (5 minutes)

Step 1: Spread oil.

Step 2: Digital-press Quchi (LI 11), Shousanli (LI 10), Hegu (LI 4) and Laogong (PC 8).

Step 3: Rub and knead the arms.

Step 4: Relax the arms.

Step 5: Lift the arms.

2.8 Massage on the anterior of the leg: Twice for each step (5 minutes)

Step 1: Spread oil.

Step 2: Digital-press Fengshi (GB 31), Xuehai (SP 10), Liangqiu (ST 34), Zusanli (ST 36), Yinlingquan (SP 9), and Sanyinjiao (SP 6).

Step 3: Push the stomach meridian of foot Yangming with the palms down, and then push the spleen meridian upward.

2.9 Shower and body care (40 minutes)

Step 1: Take a shower as required.

Step 2: Apply body mask (excluding head, face and feet), wrap in plastic wrap for 20 minutes.

Step 3: Remove the body mask.

Step 4: Apply body lotion.

Standards of working language

1. Before treatment

Hello, sir (madam)! Welcome! I'm your regulation physician. I'm very glad at your service. What we are doing today is a regulation project of medicated bath. The medicinal ingredients in the medicated bath quickly enter the body through the skin, orifices and acupoints, and with the help of heat act on the skin of the whole body, run along the meridians and collaterals and blood vessels to enter the viscera from the exterior to the interior. The combination of pushing and arc-pushing techniques along the meridians can achieve the effects of dredging meridians and collaterals, regulating yin and yang, coordinating the viscera, promoting qi and blood flow and nourishing the whole body.

Sir (madam), the treatment will take about 120 minutes. Do you need to go to the bathroom? (No.)

Do you think the light and temperature of the room are OK? (It's OK.)

Please change your clothes and take a shower first. The temperature of the medicated bath has been adjusted.

2. Treatment

Follow the steps in the treatment combined with language art.

Do you feel uncomfortable in any way? I can give you regulation based on syndrome differentiation according to your condition.

2.1 Bathing

Sir (madam), do you think the water temperature is okay? (Yes, it's good.) The bath duration is 20 minutes. If you feel unwell, please call us at any time.

Sir (madam), now I will give you a whole body massage. The massage is to press acupoints along the meridians. During the treatment, please feel the strength. If you feel unwell, please let me know.

2.2 Massage on the back

The governor vessel is the sea of yang meridians. Dredging the governor vessel can improve yang qi, prevent and improve symptoms of aversion to cold, cold hands and feet due to yang deficiency. Each five zang-organ and six fu-organ has a pair of corresponding Back-Shu acupoints on the bladder meridians. The abnormal reaction of the Back-Shu acupoint can reflect the states of the viscera. Local regulation through syndrome differentiation can achieve the overall regulation effects. The bladder meridian is also the body's defensive barrier, and enhancement of its function can help defend against wind, cold, summer-heat, dampness, dryness, fire and effectively improve the body's healthy qi and immunity. Dredging the shoulders, neck, waist and back can improve various discomforts caused by strain on the shoulder, neck, waist and back.

2.3 Massage on the buttocks

It can smooth the blood vessels and improve blood circulation in the buttocks.

2.4 Massage on the posterior of the legs

It can promote blood circulation in the legs and relieve muscular fatigue.

2.5 Massage on the chest

According to the relationship of the meridians in Chinese Medicine, the nipple belongs to the liver, and the breasts belong to the stomach. Chronic illness, physical weakness, overwork, or irregular diet can damage the spleen and stomach, cause insufficient source of qi and blood production and deplete nutrition source for the breast. Massage on Danzhong (RN 17), Rugen (ST 18) and Zusanli (ST 36) can help stimulate the liver and stomach meridians, soothe the liver and replenish blood, nourish and protect qi and blood in the breast. Adequate qi and blood can improve symptoms of fatigue, loss of appetite, abdominal distension, dizziness, vertigo, pale complexion due to qi and blood deficiency. Frequent massage on Neiguan (PC 6), Geshu (BL 17) and Ganshu (BL 18) can improve the symptoms due to liver depression and qi stagnation, such as hypochondriac distending pain, mental depression, breast distension and pain.

2.6 Massage on the abdomen

Kneading and pressing the meridians and acupoints on the abdomen can promote gastrointestinal peristalsis and excretion of the waste and turbid gas. For constipation and abdominal distension caused by poor gastrointestinal function, and distension and cold pain of the lower abdomen caused by block of the conception vessel, it has good regulating effect. And frequent massage on the abdomen can enhance fat metabolism in the abdominal region, which has the effect of weight loss.

2.7 Massage on the arms

It can enhance local blood circulation and relieve muscle pain in the arms.

2.8 Massage on the anterior of the legs

Massage on the limbs along the meridians and pressing acupoints can regulate the functions of the viscera. Simultaneously, it can dredge the meridians, promote local blood circulation, effectively enhance muscle strength and flexibility of the joint and ligament, and enhance the coordination of the limbs. It is also conducive to fat burning and plays a role in weight loss.

Breaking wind or increased urination during or after operation are normal phenomena.

3. Concluding remarks

Sir (madam), the regulation project of medicated bath has been completed. Thanks for your active cooperation. If you have any comments or suggestions, please let us know and we will definitely improve. This project is recommended to be done once a week, and I'm looking forward to seeing you next time.

Cautions

The bath water temperature is preferably 38℃ .

Pay attention to the room temperature during operation to prevent the patient from catching cold.

Final treatment

1. Patient

At the end of the treatment, the patient should be instructed to avoid exposure to coldness, drink more warm boiled water, and refrain from strenuous exercise that day. After arranging the clothes and belongings, the patient should be led to the resting place to rest for 5-10 minutes and drink 1 cup of warm boiled water or health-preserving tea.

2. Arrangement of the flexible operating table and items

Clean the flexible operating table and place it in the specified location of the treatment room.

Tidy the room and bed unit.

After the patient leaves, drain the water, disinfect the medicine bath tub, wipe the residual disinfectant, and dry it for later use.

Emergency plan

1. Allergy to medicated bath

If the patient is allergic to medicated bath, stop using the medical liquid immediately. For mild allergy, wash the affected area with warm water; for severe allergy, give anti-allergic treatment.

2. Syncope due to medicated bath

For syncope due to medicated bath with symptoms of dizziness and nausea, let the patient go out of the bath immediately and lie down, give glucose solution or normal saline orally. Open the window for ventilation and wait for the patient to stabilize. If it is not relieved, see a doctor immediately.

Knowledge reserve (knowledge related to the procedure)

1. Level 1 knowledge reserve

The understanding of the holistic concept of Chinese Medicine and the importance of regulation by medicated bath with Chinese medicine.

The function of the bladder meridian.

The function of the belt vessel.

The principle and function of aromatherapy and medicated bath.

The function of music therapy.

2. Attached formulas

Qi-Benefiting and Fatigue-Relieving Formula (Huangqi Jianzhong Decoction):

Huangqi (Radix Astragali), Guizhi (Ramulus Cinnamomi), Baishao (Radix Paeoniae Alba), Shengjiang (Rhizoma Zingiberis Recens), Dazao (Fructus Jujubae), Zhigancao (Radix et Rhizoma Glycyrrhizae Praeparata cum Melle), Dangshen (Radix Codonopsis).

Shoulder-Relaxing and Spasm-Relieving Formula (Body Pain and Stasis Expelling Decoction):

Taoren (Semen Persicae), Danggui (Radix Angelicae Sinensis), Chuanxiong (Rhizoma Chuanxiong), Qinjiao (Radix Gentianae Macrophyllae), Gancao (Radix et Rhizoma Glycyrrhizae), Yanhusuo (Rhizoma Corydalis), Qianghuo (Rhizoma et Radix Notopterygii), Moyao (Myrrha), Xiangfu (Rhizoma Cyperi) and Niuxi (Radix Achyranthis Bidentatae).

Uterus-Warming and Cold-Dissipating Formula (Mugwort and Cyperus Uterus-Warming Pill) :

Aiye (Artemisiae Argyi, Folium), Xiangfu (Rhizoma Cyperi), Wuzhuyu (Fructus Evodiae), Rougui (Cortex Cinnamomi), Danggui (Radix Angelicae Sinensis), Chuanxiong (Rhizoma Chuanxiong), Baishao (Radix Paeoniae Alba), Dihuang (Radix Rehmanniae), Huangqi (Radix Astragali), Xuduan (Radix Dipsaci).

Liver-Soothing and Depression-Relieving Formula (Chaihu Liver-Soothing Powder):

Chaihu (Radix Bupleuri), Baishao (Radix Paeoniae Alba), Zhishi (Fructus Aurantii Immaturus), Gancao (Radix et Rhizoma Glycyrrhizae), Chenpi (Pericarpium Citri Reticulatae), Xiangfu (Rhizoma Cyperi), Chuanxiong (Rhizoma Chuanxiong).

Heart-Nourishing and Mind-Tranquilizing Formula:

Guipi Decoction (used for syndrome of qi and blood deficiency):

Dangshen (Radix Codonopsis), Baizhu (Rhizoma Atractylodis Macrocephalae), Huangqi (Radix Astragali), Danggui (Radix Angelicae Sinensis), Gancao (Radix et Rhizoma Glycyrrhizae), Fushen (Sclerotium Poriae Pararadicis), Yuanzhi (Radix Polygalae), Suanzaoren (Semen Ziziphi Spinosae), Muxiang (Radix Aucklandiae), Longyanrou (Arillus Longan), Shengjiang (Rhizoma Zingiberis Recens), Dazao (Fructus Jujubae).

Suanzaoren Decoction (for syndrome of yin and blood deficiency):

Chuanxiong (Rhizoma Chuanxiong), Zhimu (Rhizoma Anemarrhenae), Fushen (Sclerotium Poriae Pararadicis), Gancao (Radix et Rhizoma Glycyrrhizae), Suanzaoren (Semen Ziziphi Spinosae).

Evaluation standards of the techniques for the operation of regulation with medicated bath

See the table below for the evaluation standards of the techniques for the operation of regulation with medicated bath.

Evaluation standards of the techniques for the operation of regulation with medicated bath

Total score of the project (100 points)	Requirements	Score	Evaluation description	Deduction
Quality requirements (5 points)	Presentable appearance, elegant manner, amiable attitude, neat clothes, hand washing, mask wearing.	5	Points will be deducted as appropriate according to the completion condition.	

Total score of the project (100 points)		Requirements	Score	Evaluation description	Deduction
Pre-operation preparation (25 points)	Notification	Time required for treatment, effects, techniques, possible local symptoms, obtaining of patient's cooperation.	4	Points will be deducted as appropriate according to condition of notification.	
	Evaluation	(Four diagnostic methods) present history, past history, family history, history of allergies, pregnancy or menstrual period; skin condition of the operation region, tolerance to pain, etc.	10	Points will be deducted as appropriate according to the evaluation condition.	
	Items	1 flexible operating table. The upper layer: 1 bottle of Collateral-Dredging Oil (10-30ml), 1 bottle of shower gel, 1 bottle of shampoo, 1 aroma lamp, 1 music player, 1 disposable medicated bath cover, 1 body mask, 1 bottle of body lotion. The lower layer: 1 shower cap, 1 bed sheet, 2 bath towels, 2 towels (30 cm × 70 cm), 2 disposable underwear, and health-preserving clothes.	5	Points will be deducted as appropriate according to the condition of imperfect item preparation.	

Continued

Total score of the project (100 points)		Requirements	Score	Evaluation description	Deduction
Pre-operation preparation (25 points)	Patients and environment	Ask the patient about preparations before treatment, take a reasonable position, and loosen clothes. Keep the room tidy, protect privacy, keep warm and avoid convection wind.	6	3 points for each of the two items. Points will be deducted as appropriate if the answer is not perfect.	
Process of the operation (40 points)	Check the doctor's advice	Check the name and diagnosis, etc.	3	3 points will be deducted if check is not performed; points will be deducted as appropriate for incomplete contents.	
	Operation	Operate in accordance with the standard technical operating procedures (steps are attached, write the scores in detail).	25	Score according to the detailed points after the table.	
	Observation	During the treatment, ask the patient about his or her feelings; comfort level and condition of pain;observe the skin condition of the operation region.	7	7 points will be deducted for failure to communicate with the patient, and points will be deducted as appropriate for incomplete contents.	

Total score of the project (100 points)		Requirements	Score	Evaluation description	Deduction
Process of the operation (40 points)	After treatment	Ask the patient about his or her feelings and inform relevant precautions; assist the patient to take a comfortable position.	5	3 points will be deducted for failure to inform, and 2 points will be deducted for failure to arrange the patient's position.	
Post-operation (20 points)	Arrangement	Make up the bed unit, arrange things, clean and disinfect the items and put them in the original places, wash hands.	5	Points will be deducted as appropriate if the arrangement is not complete.	
	Evaluation	The operation part is accurate, the manipulation is skillful, the communication with the patient is good, and the patient feels that the expected goal is achieved.	5	Points will be deducted as appropriate if the evaluation is not complete.	
	Medical record	Detailed medical records to record treatment conditions, signature.	2	2 points will be deducted for failure to record; 1 point will be deducted for incomplete records.	

Continued

Total score of the project (100 points)		Requirements	Score	Evaluation description	Deduction
Post-operation (20 points)	Post-operation disposal	Used materials are handled in accordance with "Technical Standards for Disinfection of Medical Institutions".	8	For incorrect disposal method, 2 points will be deducted for each item.	
Theoretical questions (10 points)		Relevant knowledge of medicated bath. Precautions for the operation of medicated bath.	10	2 points will be deducted for incomplete answer of each question; 5 points will be deducted for no answer to each question.	

Total score:

Signature of the examiner: Assessment date:

Appendix with operation steps and scoring points:

1. Bathing, bath time 20 minutes (3 points)

2. Massage on the back (5 points)

Step 1: Spread oil.

Step 2: To dredge the governor vessel and overlap and rub warm the two hands.

Step 3: Push the bladder meridian and pull back the hand to the fingertips to expel toxin.

Step 4: Dredge the hypochondriac regions.

Step 5: Press Dazhui (DU 14) and the acupoints on the first lateral line of the bladder meridians on the back with both thumbs.

Step 6: Push the back in Tai Chi style.

Step 7 Digital-press Mingmen (DU 4) with both thumbs.

3. Massage on the buttocks (2 points)

Step 1: Spread oil.

Step 2: Digital-press the acupoints.

Step 3: Lift the buttocks.

Step 4: Press Huantiao (GB 30) and Chengfu (BL 36) with both thumbs.

4. Massage on the posterior of the legs (2 points)

Step 1: Spread oil.

Step 2: Digital-press Chengfu (BL 36), Weizhong (BL 40) and Chengshan (BL 57).

Step 3: Dredge the bladder meridians on the posterior part of the legs with both hands.

Step 4: Press Chengfu (BL 36), Weizhong (BL 40) and Chengshan (BL 57), grasp and knead the muscles of the calves.

5. Massage on the chest (4 points)

Step 1: Spread oil.

Step 2: Digital-press Tiantu (RN 22), Danzhong (RN 17), Rugen (ST 18), Wuyi (ST 15) and Yunmen (LU 2).

Step 3: Lift the breasts.

Step 4: To find out nodules.

Step 5: Digital-press Tiantu (RN 22), Danzhong (RN 17), Rugen (ST 18), Wuyi (ST 15) and Yunmen (LU 2).

6. Massage on the abdomen (4 points)

Step 1: Spread oil.

Step 2: Digital-press Shangwan (RN 13), Zhongwan (RN 12), Xiawan (RN 10), Qihai (RN 6) and Guanyuan (RN 4).

Step 3: Dredge the conception vessel.

Step 4: Dredge the side waist.

Step 5: Push and knead the side waist with both hands.

Step 6: Rub warm Shenque (RN 8) with both hands.

Step 7: To expel toxin.

7. Massage on the arms (3 points)

Step 1: Spread oil.

Step 2: Digital-press Quchi (LI 11), Shousanli (LI 10), Hegu (LI 4) and Laogong (PC 8).

Step 3: Rub and knead the arms.

Step 4: Relax the arms.

Step 5: Lift the arms.

8. Massage on the anterior part of the legs (2 points)

Step 1: Spread oil.

Step 2: Digital-press Fengshi (GB 31), Xuehai (SP 10), Liangqiu (ST 34), Zusanli (ST 36), Yinlingquan (SP 9), and Sanyinjiao (SP 6).

Step 3: Push the stomach meridian of foot Yangming with the palms down, and then push the spleen meridian upward.

Section 8 Moxibustion on the Governor Vessel

Name of the project

Moxibustion on the governor vessel is an external treatment in Chinese Medicine which applies indirect moxibustion to the regions of the cervical, thoracic and lumbar spine of the governor vessel to prevent and cure diseases and strengthen the body.

The function of the project

It has the function of invigorating the kidney and dredging the governor vessel, warming yang and dissipating cold, strengthening the bones and permeating the muscles, dispelling blood stasis and eliminating stagnation, smoothing the joint and relieving pain.

Indications

It is suitable for relieving joint pains such as neck, shoulder, waist, legs and soft tissue sprains caused by wind cold and pathogenic dampness.

It is suitable for patients with symptom of aversion to cold, such as cold hands and feet, dysmenorrhea due to cold uterus.

It is suitable for diseases due to qi deficiency, chronic fatigue syndrome, poor immunity, etc.

Contraindications

Patients with serious internal diseases, or patients with pacemakers, or patients with heart decompensation should not be applied with this therapy. It is forbidden for patients with high fever or diabetes.

It is forbidden for patients with disease of bleeding tendency, local skin damage and infection, hyper-irritability.

It is forbidden for women during menstruation and pregnancy.

It is forbidden for acute injury.

The use for children must be under the supervision of adults.

Standard technical operation procedures

1. Preparations

1.1 Pre-operation preparation for the operator

The operator should perform personal hygiene (including nail cutting), disinfect hands, wear neat clothes and a mask.

Appendix 1

The preparation of ginger shreds: An appropriate amount of ginger (the rate of shredded ginger after preparation is about 55%), cut the ginger into small pieces, put it into the cooking machine, turn on the power, and break into mashed ginger. Shake the cooking machine during the mashing process to speed up the process. Take out the mashed ginger, squeeze it evenly with both hands, and squeeze out the ginger juice until there is no ginger juice flowing out when mild pressure is applied.

Appendix 2

The preparation of moxa cone: Divide 100 g moxa into five equal parts, put each part in the palm of one hand, use the other hand to press and twist to form oval or long strips of about 5 cm in length. The tighter the better. It is advisable that the moxa will not scatter when placed.

1.2 Items preparation

1 flexible operating table. ① The upper layer: Take 1 ware of suitable size to prepare 700g (for women) or 800g (for men) of mashed ginger, 75% alcohol cotton ball, 5 moxa cone, 1 alcohol lamp, 1 lighter, 1 joss-stick, 1 moxibustion device for the governor vessel. ② The lower layer: 1 bed sheet, 2 towels (30 cm × 70 cm), 1 bath towel and health-preserving clothes. ③ The tools used for moxibustion on the governor vessel should be made of solid wood whose heat insulation is relatively stable. Please refer to the figure below for the selection of specific size.

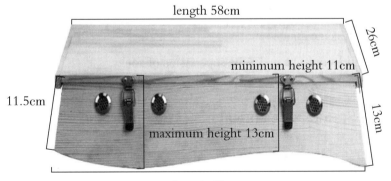

length 58cm

26cm

minimum height 11cm

11.5cm

13cm

maximum height 13cm

length 60cm

1.3 Preparation of the patient

Put on health-preserving clothes, lay prone on the treatment bed, expose Dazhui (DU 14) on the back to the region of Baliao acupoints, and place the upper limbs on both sides of the body.

2. Operation

Step 1: Disinfection. Routinely disinfect 3 times along the spine with 75% alcohol cotton balls from top to bottom. (3 minutes)

Step 2: Place the moxa cones. Place the 5 moxa cones in the device for moxibustion on the governor vessel and lay them up and down one by one. (2 minutes)

Step 3: Location. Place the device for moxibustion on the governor vessel on the spine from Dazhui (DU 14) to Baliao acupoints. (1 minute)

Step 4: Ignition. Use the joss-stick to light the two ends of the moxa cones from bottom to top. (3 minutes)

Step 5: Control the temperature. Time the moxibustion since it starts. Ask the patient how the temperature feels about 20 minutes after the application of moxibustion (usually the temperature will reach the highest after 20 minutes) and whether there is any burning sensation. If the patient feels hot obviously, immediately remove the device, place it in a clean place and quickly spread the sterilized towel on the region with hot sensation, and then place the moxibustion box well again. After about 5 minutes, ask the patient again how he feels. After 35 minutes of moxibustion, ask the patient about the temperature. If the temperature drops slightly, take off the towel and continue moxibustion for 10 minutes to end the moxibustion. (50 minutes)

Step 6: After the operation, remove the device, clean the sweat and ginger juice on the patient's back. (1 minute)

Standards of working language

1. Before treatment

Hello, sir (madam)! Welcome! I am your regulation physician. I'm very happy to be at your service. What we are doing today is the project of moxibustion on the governor vessel. It has the effects of invigorating the kidney and dredging the governor vessel, warming yang and dissipating cold, strengthening the bones and permeating the muscles, dispelling blood stasis and eliminating stagnation, smoothing the joint and relieving pain.

The treatment duration is about 60 minutes. Do you need to go to the bathroom? (No.)

Sir (madam), please take off your coat, and I will help you hang it on the hanger. First, please take a prone position on this bed.

2. Treatment

Follow the steps in the treatment combined with language art.

Step 1: Disinfection. Hello, sir (madam)! According to your treatment needs, I will disinfect your moxibustion site now. As alcohol is used, it will be slightly irritate to the skin, please endure the pain a little.

Step 2: Place the moxibustion box.

Step 3: Location. Sir (madam), I'm applying moxibustion on the acupoints of the governor vessel on the back. All of the governor vessel, conception vessel and thoroughfare vessel start from the uterus. The governor vessel runs on the region of the waist and back while the conception vessel and thoroughfare vessel run on the regions of the chest and abdomen. The governor vessel is the sea of yang vessel, governing various yang of the body. Yin meridians converge at the yang meridians through the meridian branches. Therefore, the governor vessel can connect the meridians and collaterals of the whole body. Through the comprehensive effects of moxibustion on the governor vessel to stimulate and coordinate various meridians, the meridians and collaterals can exert their functions of connecting the viscera internally, associating the limbs and joints externally, communicating the interior with the exterior, transporting qi and blood, balancing yin and yang, thus achieving the purpose of health preservation. It also plays a role in health care and health preservation for healthy people. In modern society, people are tired from long-term work, staying up late, overeating of cold food (such as frozen food in the refrigerator), and excessive use of air conditioners. These all consume the body's yang qi. People feel that their bodies are getting more and more tired, and their spirits are getting more and more depressed. These are the so-called "sub-health" states. At present, there is no specific method for these symptoms in modern medicine. However, the physical treatment and intervention method of moxibustion on the governor vessel can not only improve symptoms, but also prevent diseases and maintain health. This is also the "preventive treatment" advocated by modern society.

Step 4: Ignition. Use the joss-stick to light the two ends of the moxa cones from bottom to top. Sir (madam), I have lit the moxa cone now, and the temperature will rise slowly. If you feel hot or have other discomforts, please tell me in time.

3. Concluding remarks

Sir (madam), the treatment project of the moxibustion on the governor vessel has ended. Thanks for your active cooperation. If you have any suggestions, please let us know and we will actively improve.

Precautions

Pay attention to the room temperature and the patient should keep warm during treatment.

During moxibustion, observe the temperature at any time to avoid scalding the patient. The temperature should be comfortable for the patient and not too hot.

Elderly patients should not lie prone for too long, and the treatment time can be shortened appropriately.

Ask the patient not to take a bath within 6 hours after treatment.

Final treatment

1. Patient

After the treatment, the sweat and ginger juice on the back of the patient should be wiped off. Ask the patient to avoid exposing to cold, drink more warm boiled water, and refrain from strenuous exercise that day. After the patient has arranged his or her clothes, lead him or her to the lobby to rest for 5-10 minutes and drink 1 cup of warm boiled water or health-preserving herbal tea.

2. Arrangement of the flexible operating table and items

Clean up the flexible operating table, put back all items to their original positions and the flexible operating table to the specified position in the treatment room.

Clean the inside and outside of the device for moxibustion on the governor vessel, and dry it for later use.

Tidy the room and bed unit.

Emergency plan

1. Dizziness after the treatment

A few patients will experience dizziness after treatment, which is caused by a sudden change in body position. Give proper glucose solution orally and ask the patient to lie on the back to rest for a while. If it is not relieved, give corresponding treatment. Ask a senior physician for guidance if necessary.

2. Blisters due to moxibustion

Refer to the cupping treatment method in the first section of this chapter "Spinal Regulation".

Knowledge reserve (knowledge related to the procedure)

Level 1 knowledge reserve

The understanding of the holistic concept of Chinese Medicine and the importance of regulation of the back.

The running route of the governor vessel, location of key acupoints and their indications.

The location and indications of Jiaji (EX-B2).

The basic content of yin and yang theory and its application in Chinese Medicine.

Evaluation standards of the techniques for the operation of moxibustion on the governor vessel

See the table below for the evaluation standards of the techniques for the operation of moxibustion on the governor vessel.

Evaluation standards of the techniques for the operation of moxibustion on the governor vessel

Total score of the project (100 points)		Requirements	Score	Evaluation description	Deduction
Quality requirements (5 points)		Presentable appearance, elegant manner, amiable attitude, neat clothes, hand washing, mask wearing.	5	Points will be deducted as appropriate according to the completion condition.	
Pre-operation preparation (25 points)	Notification	Time required for treatment, effects, techniques, possible local symptoms, obtaining of patient's cooperation.	4	Points will be deducted as appropriate according to condition of notification.	
	Evaluation	(Four diagnostic methods) present history, past history, family history, history of allergies, pregnancy or menstrual period; skin condition of the operation region, tolerance to pain, etc.	10	Points will be deducted as appropriate according to the evaluation condition.	

Continued

Total score of the project (100 points)		Requirements	Score	Evaluation description	Deduction
Pre-operation preparation (25 points)	Items	1 flexible operating table. The upper layer: 1 utensil, 700 g of shredded ginger (women), 800 g (men), 75% alcohol cotton balls, 5 moxa cones, 1 alcohol lamp, 1 lighter, 1 joss-stick, 1 apparatus for moxibustion on the governor vessel The lower layer: 1 bed sheet, 2 towels (30 cm× 70 cm), 1 bath towel and health-preserving clothes.	5	Points will be deducted as appropriate according to the condition of imperfect item preparation.	
	Patients and environment	Ask the patient about preparations before treatment, take a reasonable position, and loosen clothes. Keep the room tidy, protect privacy, keep warm and avoid convection wind.	6	3 points for each of the two items. Points will be deducted as appropriate if the answer is not perfect.	
Process of the operation (40 points)	Check the doctor's advice	Check the name and diagnosis, etc.	3	3 points will be deducted if check is not performed; points will be deducted as appropriate for incomplete contents.	

Total score of the project (100 points)		Requirements	Score	Evaluation description	Deduction
Process of the operation (40 points)	Operation	Operate in accordance with the standard technical operating procedures (steps are attached, write the scores in detail).	25	Score according to the detailed points after the table.	
	Observation	During the treatment, ask the patient about his or her feelings; comfort level and condition of pain;observe the skin condition of the operation region.	7	7 points will be deducted for failure to communicate with the patient, and points will be deducted as appropriate for incomplete contents.	
	After treatment	Ask the patient about his or her feelings and inform relevant precautions; assist the patient to take a comfortable position.	5	3 points will be deducted for failure to inform, and 2 points will be deducted for failure to arrange the patient's position.	
Post-operation (20 points)	Arrangement	Make up the bed unit, arrange things, clean and disinfect the items and put them in the original places, wash hands.	5	Points will be deducted as appropriate if the arrangement is not complete.	

Continued

Total score of the project (100 points)		Requirements	Score	Evaluation description	Deduction
Post-operation (20 points)	Evaluation	The operation part is accurate, the manipulation is skillful, the communication with the patient is good, the patient feels that the expected goal is achieved.	5	Points will be deducted as appropriate if the evaluation is not complete.	
	Medical record	Detailed medical records to record treatment conditions, signature.	2	2 points will be deducted for failure to record; 1 point will be deducted for incomplete records.	
	Post-operation disposal	Used materials are handled in accordance with "Technical Standards for Disinfection of Medical Institutions".	8	For incorrect disposal method, 2 points will be deducted for each item.	

Total score of the project (100 points)	Requirements	Score	Evaluation description	Deduction
Theoretical questions (10 points)	Relevant knowledge of moxibustion on the governor vessel. Operation precautions of the moxibustion on the governor vessel.	10	2 points will be deducted for incomplete answer of each question; 5 points will be deducted for no answer to each question.	

Total score:

Signature of the examiner: Assessment date:

Appendix with operation steps and scoring points:

Step 1: Disinfection. (4 points)

Step 2: Place the moxa cones. (4 points)

Step 3: Location. (4 points)

Step 4: Ignition. (4 points)

Step 5: Control the temperature. (7 points)

Step 6: After the operation, remove the device, clean the sweat and ginger juice on the patient's back.(2 minutes)